Dustin Peone

Literary Meditations for Pandemic Times

Reflections on Plague Classics

STUDIES IN MEDICAL PHILOSOPHY

Edited by Alexander Gungov and Friedrich Luft

ISSN 2367-4377

1 *David Låg Tomasi*
Medical Philosophy
A Philosophical Analysis of Patient Self-Perception in Diagnostics and Therapy
ISBN 978-3-8382-0935-7

2 *Jean Buttigieg*
The Human Genome as Common Heritage of Mankind
ISBN 978-3-8382-1157-2

3 *Donald Phillip Verene*
The Science of Cookery and the Art of Eating Well
Philosophical and Historical Reflections on Food and Dining in Culture
ISBN 978-3-8382-1198-5

4 *Jean-Pierre Clero*
Rethinking Medical Ethics
Concepts and Principles
ISBN 978-3-8382-1194-7

5 *Alexander L. Gungov*
Patient Safety
The Relevance of Logic in Medical Care
ISBN 978-3-8382-1213-5

6 *Ken A. Bryson*
A Systems Analysis of Medicine (SAM)
Healing Medicine
ISBN 978-3-8382-1267-8

7 *Dmitry A. Balalykin*
Galen on Apodictics
ISBN 978-3-8382-1406-1

8 *Raymond C. Barfield*
The Practice of Medicine as Being in Time
ISBN 978-3-8382-1427-6

9 *Dustin Peone*
Literary Meditations for Pandemic Times
Reflections on Plague Classics
ISBN 978-3-8382-1756-7

Dustin Peone

LITERARY MEDITATIONS FOR PANDEMIC TIMES

Reflections on Plague Classics

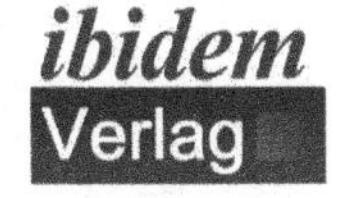

Bibliographic information published by the Deutsche Nationalbibliothek
Die Deutsche Nationalbibliothek lists this publication in the Deutsche Nationalbibliografie; detailed bibliographic data are available in the Internet at http://dnb.d-nb.de.

Bibliografische Information der Deutschen Nationalbibliothek
Die Deutsche Nationalbibliothek verzeichnet diese Publikation in der Deutschen Nationalbibliografie; detaillierte bibliografische Daten sind im Internet über http://dnb.d-nb.de abrufbar.

Cover illustration: *Music*, © copyright 2020 by Megan Lillie

First edition published as *Plague Literature: Lessons for Living Well during a Pandemic*. Atlanta: Theuth Books, 2020.

ISBN-13: 978-3-8382-1756-7

Printed in the United States of America

For all nurses,
especially Erin Peone,
Kelsey Esch,
Lindsay Lana,
and Billy Wolfe.

“Weak as I am, I carry on the war to the last moment, I get a hundred pike-thrusts, I return two hundred, and I laugh. I see near my door Geneva on fire with quarrels over nothing, and I laugh again; and, thank God, I can look upon the world as a farce even when it becomes as tragic as it sometimes does. All comes out even at the end of the day, and all comes out still more even when all the days are over.”

—Voltaire

CONTENTS

Preface to the Second Edition

At present, it is two years and several months since the start of the COVID-19 pandemic. In anthropomorphic terms, our worldwide crisis is now a toddler. It no longer requires our constant attention and vigilance, and our thoughts are finally able to expand beyond the basic concern of survival. However, the toddler does not yet cease to tyrannize. At times of calm, it screams for attention. It acts out and breaks something once in a while. We are close to resuming some semblance of normalcy, but COVID continues to surprise us.

Less significantly, it is now nearly two years since the first publication of my book, *Plague Literature: Lessons for Living Well during a Pandemic.*[1] It pleases me immensely that after all this time, and in spite of the inverted world in which we have abided, there remains an audience for this little tome. It is republished here with a new title, but substantially unchanged, save for minor copyediting and typesetting corrections. To introduce the book to new readers, it seems proper to say something about its origin and composition, as well as its reception. Also, having written the book during the first act of the COVID pandemic, it will be worthwhile to reflect on this modern plague from the point of view of the fifth act.

In the fateful month of March, 2020, I was lecturing at Oglethorpe University. Like most of academia, I found myself, without much preparation, having to transition all of my classes into remote learning. There are fields of study in which little is lost by this transition, but philosophy, which since Socrates has been rooted in conversation, is not among these. The pedagogical disadvantages of remote education compelled me to supplement my lectures with a series of podcasts made for my classes. Each week, I would interview two or three scholars from around the country, and engage in philosophical discussions on topics of their choosing. Some of these discussions were deeply serious, others delightfully whimsical. My guiding principle was, since the students could no longer be involved in classroom conversation, to continue to expose them to the great conversation of ideas that never ends.

From the start, these conversations tended to literary, and my interlocutors and I would discuss what books we were reading for edification. Many of the scholars I spoke with said that they were reading a great deal of Scripture, for spiritual consolation—this was true of both believers and

1 First edition: Atlanta: Theuth Books, 2020.

non-believers. Many also said that they found themselves better able to orient to the ongoing situation by reading the classic works of plague literature. Most frequently, it was Camus to whom they turned; occasionally, Daniel Defoe. Gregory McBrayer said that he had been reading Strozzi and Machiavelli's "Epistle"; my thanks are due to him for introducing me to this odd document. Kafka also figured into many conversations, as one might expect any time the human condition is existentially threatened.

These books are not self-help books or programs of amelioration. They do not tell us how to end pandemics or treat the infected. The technicians involved with synthesizing vaccinations or emergency civic planning are not (and should not be) looking to Camus to tell them their business. These books are not by any means *solutions*; they are literature. That does not mean, however, that they yield no benefit. Literature helps us because it gives us insight into the souls of others. Descartes says, "Reading good books is like having a conversation with the most distinguished men of past ages—indeed, a rehearsed conversation in which these authors reveal to us only the best of their thoughts."[2] Descartes was, in general, a despiser of classical education, but he still recognized this fundamental truth. We continue to read classic works because they continue to speak to us today, and their speech is living. Books whose speech is dead to us are preserved only on the dusty shelves of philologists.

Scholars have a broader experience in reading great literature than the average layperson (*nota bene*, this does not mean that they are better readers). The idea of picking up Camus during a contemporary plague is one of the earliest thoughts of most academic professors. Camus' *Plague* is not, however, common currency amongst laypersons. It struck me that some good might be done if a scholar were to write a philosophical book for an audience wider than academia, meditating upon the insights of the great writers of the past concerning pandemics. Such a book could point the reader to a syllabus of rewarding classic books on the topic. It could also, by contemplating the central ideas of these books, offer spiritual solace in its own right. This thought was at the genesis of the present volume.

Once conceived, the first edition wrote itself in a matter of weeks. Wilhelm Dilthey observes, "It seems to have been one of the accepted

2 René Descartes, *Discourse on Method*, in *The Philosophical Writings of Descartes*, vol. 1, trans. John Cottingham, Robert Stoothoff, and Dugald Murdoch (New York: Cambridge University Press, 1997), Part One, 113.

principles of ancient poetics that poetic creativity was a kind of madness."[3] The writer's art has always been psychologically akin to frenzy. The composition of this book was no exception, composed in the midst of *furia eroica*. I meditated upon books I loved, and—in common with the rest of the world at that time—I had plenty of time for meditation. The result is before you. It is not a treatise and it contains little or no argument. Properly speaking, this book is in the literary tradition of *pensées*. The chapters of this volume are a gathering of thoughts, not parts of a complex sorities. The spirit of the work is contemplative, not apodictic, just as the works of which it treats were composed in the spirit of contemplation. My various reflections are so many offerings for the human spirit. They will yield much more if approached with a sense of wonder and imagination than if approached with a sense of calculative pragmatism.

The response to this book has surprised me. It has received little attention from the philosophical community at large, but this was not unexpected. Philosophers are all solipsists, disinterested in whatever they themselves have not created. The average professional philosopher reminds one of Beckett's great character Murphy, who has a mind like "a large hollow sphere, hermetically closed to the universe without."[4] What was unexpected was the positive feedback my book received from the medical community.

In the book's introduction, I wrote, "It is the physician's work to treat the body during this pandemic. … However, the human being is more than so many pounds of flesh. The human being is a creature with an inner life as well as an epidermis. The question of *how to live well during a pandemic* is not a question for [physicians and other experts]." I did not intend this or other passages as a denigration of medicine (though at times I am critical of medical *rhetoric*, which is a different matter). My purpose was to offer these literary meditations as a supplement to medical intervention, not a replacement. The physicians are the proper healers of the body, but poetic wisdom is the best medicine for the soul. During a medical crisis, both aspects of the human self, body and spirit, come under duress and require thoughtful care. Medicine and the humanities are called to work hand in hand. This is a view that goes back at least to Plato.

---

3 Wilhelm Dilthey, "The Imagination of the Poet," in *Selected Works, vol. 5: Poetry and Experience*, ed. Rudolf A Makkreel and Frithjof Rodi (Princeton, NJ: Princeton University Press, 1985), 67.

4 Samuel Beckett, *Murphy* (New York: Grove Press, 1957), 65.

My intention was never to offer guidance to the medical community itself. What could a speculative dreamer have to teach to a healer of the flesh? Socrates piously sacrifices to Asclepius, and never seeks to instruct the god. Nevertheless, it has been my great and unforeseen honor to be widely accepted by medical professionals. I know of a hospital chaplain who has quoted from the book in her sermons. I have been told by several nurses that they read the text to some profit. I even learned that the book has been used for two semesters as a textbook for Duke University medical students. When I met with those classes, led by Brian Quaranta and Jehanne Gheith, and sponsored by Duke's Trent Center for Bioethics, Humanities, and History of Medicine, I found a welcoming and receptive audience. My experience has led me to believe that there is more space for—and interest in—productive collaboration between medicine and the humanities than one might imagine. The two fields can do more than supplement each other; they can actively inform one another.

The negative feedback that the book has received has taken the form of a defense of medicine against my ruminations. The curiosity is that this criticism has come from within the humanities, *not* within the medical sphere. As a representative example of the misunderstandings of critics with regard to my purpose, I will point the reader to a review of the book in *Rain Taxi Review of Books*, by Mr. John Toren.[5] This dyspeptic review has nothing positive whatsoever to say about *Plague Literature*. These are Mr. Toren's primary criticisms:

(1) I reject medical science in favor of literary rumination and poetic "folk-doctoring." (2) My style is "scattershot and digressive," the trains of thought "erratic," and their interpenetration "rare." (3) Most damningly, I do not adequately engage with the texts by way of the accepted modes of literary criticism. I take what I want from them like a succubus, and then cast them aside for my own meandering disquisitions.

(1) The first criticism is politically motivated, and is perhaps the real axe that Mr. Toren has to grind. He forgets, though, the context and time of my writing. I was not responding to a pandemic in full swing, nor belittling the evidence-based recommendations of the medical community that began to be circulated after we had been dealing with COVID for half a year. The fact that "in many areas of the country the practice [of social distancing] has been widely ignored for months" is a commonplace observation, but here irrelevant. I was not writing *after* those "months," but before them. When I composed, the medical community had little to offer in

5 *Rain Taxi Review of Books* 26, no. 2 (Summer 2021): 31.

the way of health procedures, and "social distancing" was all one heard about. I still maintain, as I say in the text, that this notion was ill-conceived, poorly worded, and foisted upon us as though it was a cure-all. Mr. Toren presents it as a "fact" that no one promoted it in these terms. Very well, but am I mistaken about the *spirit* in which it was promoted in those early days? Were we not told by every talking head that the pandemic would be a short-term affair, which we could avoid by simply giving others a bit of space and keeping our hands clean? Even the appropriateness of masking came as a late discovery. Mr. Toren intimates that I am an anti-masker or an anti-vaccer, or the voice of some other counter-cultural political interest, contrasting my "pre-scientific" insights with "masks, vaccines, social distancing," and so on. I am none of those things, but more significantly, as I wrote, those categories did not yet exist.

I have heard a few others voice concerns that I seem to undermine medical prescriptions. I will not venture an opinion as to whether the CDC and other health organizations have come through the pandemic with their reputations intact; I leave this critique for others. I will, however, say that I know of no person working in the medical field who has made the mistake of thinking that I claim to offer literary wisdom as a *substitute* for medical knowledge. I make it perfectly clear that for matters of our bodily well-being we ought to follow the dictates of the Hippocratics. My only assertion is that the poets (here, as in all life situations) can sing to us of living well, while physicians sing of living healthfully.

(2) A true believer, advocating for an ideology, has to do with argument, and argument must be concise and direct. I have never been an ideologue, and I therefore reject the notion that philosophy is equivalent to argument. I do not trade in dogmatics and, like my Italian forebears, I am at home in syncretism. Like John the Baptist, I *point*. Pointing allows the reader to partake of the intellectual journey as a fellow-traveler. I wander, I take my time here, I speed by there. On occasion, I perambulate in the gyres of Yeats. This is a matter of taste. Here, the taste of Mr. Toren and myself clash.

My "many rhetorical blunders" and "internal contradictions" (Toren's phrases) are perhaps unforgivable. Or perhaps they are stages of dialectical thinking, which Mr. Toren does not seem to consider. Where he wants analytic precision, he has stumbled into a world of Montaigne and Hegel, and he finds himself adrift. This is not at all what he hoped to find. He perhaps wanted authoritative answers, and all he finds are processes of thought. Does *he* have answers? Does he chafe just as much when he reads Montaigne's *Essais*, with their frequent turnabouts, their digressions, their many contradictions? How does he feel about Pascal's *Penseés*? How does he get through—Heaven preserve us—a reading of Joyce? I follow the thought where it leads, and my only concern is to show that progress to the reader, not to stand firm on any article of faith or other.

(3) Mr. Toren's final criticism, which he discusses at greatest length, is that I do not treat the books I use with any sort of critical method. For example, in analyzing the *Decameron*, where "we might expect Peone to provide a few examples of [Boccaccio's wit] from the tales, and then clarify how they illuminate or provide an appropriate response to the widespread suffering and death taking place in Florence. … He chooses, rather, to drop references to the *Decameron* entirely, inserting instead an abstract six-page disquisition on the nature and meaning of humor," and so on. (Incidentally, since the Boccaccio chapter is the only one about which Mr. Toren says a word, one may assume it is the only chapter he bothered to read. Imagine his disgust had he continued on!)

"In short," the critique continues, "Peone doesn't engage the text, but merely uses it as a touchstone to support a variety of seemingly random, often half-baked, and sometimes ill-informed ruminations." But this is precisely what an *assayer* does with raw ore, and what an *essayer* does with raw ideas. I eschew all schools of criticism, not because they are worthless, but because I have no interest in performing literary criticism. I do not believe I ever presented myself in such a light. What I sought to do with this volume is to think along with the great thinkers. I had no intention of doing them "justice." Their insights are those of human beings of a different time and place. I wanted to see what *we* might think when reading them today, what thoughts they might inspire and what ruminations they might instigate. I do not read literature as a scholar, but as a thinking man. That is why I continue to enjoy literature. Montaigne said of Plutarch, "I cannot be with him even a little without taking out a drumstick or a wing."[6] I, too, use my authors as nutrition. I grab a wing from Thucydides, a leg from Rabelais, a cutlet of Camus. I eat like a cow, chewing the cud. Again, Mr. Toren's conflict with me is merely a matter of taste. Toren says that I am not "the right man for the job." Certainly not, but only because he and I differ as to what the job actually is. Mr. Toren would prefer I make gizmos, and I have made widgets instead. He cares about the books I reflect upon

6 Michel de Montaigne, *The Complete Essays of Montaigne*, trans. Donald M. Frame (Stanford, CA: Stanford University Press, 1976), 666.

as ends in themselves. Every good book is an end in itself, but it is also a means, and that is how I have used literature here.

Enough of this. Responding to one's critics is futile, and keeps their criticism alive long past its due. (Would anyone today have heard of Rodbertus had Engels not devoted so much effort to refuting his accusations against Marx?) I prefer to believe that, after my *apologia*, Mr. Toren and I, like Socrates and Thrasymachus, are now friends. I ought to have warned the reader from the start of the first volume that he or she would not be opening a book of literary criticism of an approved style. I have amended this by amending the book's title. *Literary Meditations for Pandemic Times: Reflections on Plague Classics*. There can now be no mistaking the nature of the book. Herein are meditations, ruminations, reflections. These are dialectical essays, not arguments. They are the expression of living thought, grappling with the unknown. They perambulate through the fine summer air breathed by literary giants. I have no answers for sale, but my hope is that these ruminations might inspire some readers to reflect on these weighty matters for themselves and to turn to the books I discuss as "touchstones" of their own.

These meditations were first offered up at a time when no such book existed, when people were in need of a polestar by which to orient their lives. I offer them again to a new people, a people that has largely come through crisis and has learned much by its own lights. We are no longer who we were. In some instances, the observations I make are specific to our situation from early 2020. On the whole, though, having read through the volume once more, I find that much of what I have said is relevant to dark times in general. My epigraph, from Voltaire, was chosen not because it has any particular relevance to COVID-19 but because it is mankind's proper mantra for dark times.

To revise my essays in light of what we have learned over the last two years would be to write an entirely new work, which other obligations—and a disinclination to tread the same ground twice—prevent me from attempting. Other books in a similar vein have sprung up since the first edition of this book was published, and bourgeois journals have abounded with articles on the topic, which makes me feel that it is no longer a pressing duty for me to continue my task. I will, however, say a few words about the past two years. In particular, I will briefly indicate the two phenomena that I believe have been most philosophically significant over this time, one social, the other psychological. These two phenomena ought to inform the trends of research in the social sciences for the near future.

In face of the pandemic, the world suffered an intense strain on all social institutions. Financial systems, educational systems, political systems, criminal justice systems, healthcare systems, and so forth all depend upon a certain regularity of conditions. During a crisis, human behavior becomes highly unpredictable and erratic, which destabilizes these conditions. This destabilization tests all aspects of an institution, and throws into relief every weak point and every fissure. There is some flaw in every golden bowl. In America, everyone will recall the baffling early absence of toilet paper, the stasis period when education simply ceased, and the wildly self-contradictory statements made by health organizations. The sporadic rioting of both the left and the right during the pandemic has ostensibly had political motives, but has been hastened by a psychological need for catharsis during a period of crisis. Our politicians, our leaders, have shown themselves to be purely reactionary, with nothing at all of the great statesman in them. Great tragedies could be written about *individuals* suffering through the COVID years by our modern Aeschyluses and Euripideses, but a drama about our *institutions* could only be a comedy. Aristophanes would delight in the sheer human folly on display in the highest forums.

This uncovering of all of the shortcomings of our most enduring institutions has been brutal and dehumanizing, but it is also potentially for the good. We now know what is hidden beneath the veil of Isis. We can work to ameliorate these flaws and to improve our systems. We are called to this work, because we are aware that this crisis will not be the last we face, and how we come through the next will largely depend on how we amend those institutions that failed us on the present occasion. I say we *can* ameliorate our weaknesses, but will we? Even now, our energy for the task ebbs, and things begin to return to the status quo. Our minds and spirits are exhausted, and no one can blame anyone else for embracing the normal rather than striving for an ideal.

On a psychological level, the pandemic has made the world more protestant. There is always chatter about the virus "bringing people together," "making communities stronger," and so on, and in isolated cases, this is true. However, I do not see that the overall effect of the pandemic has been catholicizing. On the whole, amongst the working classes, the young, the old, the masses, these years have been marked by extreme social isolation. (My warning about the slogan "social distancing" was that its propagation would tend to alienate human beings from one another on a social level rather than serving its purpose, *physical* distancing.) We have been thrown upon our own resources and our own counsel, while we have been isolated from outside human contact. Many persons spent weeks at a time alone in small domiciles without venturing outside, and most of these had no previous experience of solitude. On the occasions when people dared to come together, the repressed human passions gave an orgiastic turn to their gatherings. Then, leaving the house, every social encounter was fraught. When I meet The Other in a public space, he seems to be my enemy. If he sniffles, it is a moral vice; if he coughs, it is an act of violence.

If it turns out that this crucible has made us stronger and more resilient as a species, all the better. The danger, of course, is that it has left us stunted and crippled. As we begin to return to the old ways and enter once more into the civilized world, what awaits us? Is it a city of new, higher human beings, who have made great strides in self-knowledge? Or is it Eliot's "unreal city," in which hollow men and hollow women pass us by like automata? I observe something of both when I wander about, and I do not yet know which group will come to rule the day tomorrow.

Is there more to say? There is much more to say, an endless verbiage that threatens to spill forth like froth from a chalice, but this is not the place. It behooves me now only to wish the reader well, and to encourage healthful practices for the body and literary meditations for the mind. Take my ruminations for what they are worth to you, and enjoy from my writing here a drumstick and there a wing!

Atlanta, Georgia
5 October 2022

Introduction

Looking Backward from a Pandemic

As I write this book, in the spring of 2020,[1] the factor that most dominates all social, political, and economic affairs the world over is the ongoing COVID-19 pandemic. Governments and institutions have responded to this situation in different manners, with more or less swiftness and more or less rigor. The pandemic has ravaged nations indiscriminately, beginning in Asia and moving rapidly westward. In America, now more than three months into a national outbreak, politicians and public health leaders remain without consensus about the optimal means of confronting this disease. There is no doubt that the technicians will produce a vaccine, but this prospect remains distant. In the meanwhile, common wisdom tells us that the best thing to do is to shelter ourselves in place, keep our hands washed, and practice "social distancing." What we are not told is how we ought to live and act.

"Common wisdom" is no wisdom at all, and when the solution in which we invest our faith and hope is analyzed, it reveals its inherent nothingness. The neologism "social distancing" conveys the very opposite of what it intends. This slipshod use of language will have harmful psychological consequences at some point in the near future. Those who use this term as a call to action mean to say that individuals should *physically* distance themselves one from another when in public space. The beginning student of political science has sense enough to feel that "social distancing" taken literally is an instrument of tyranny. To distance oneself socially from others is to disrupt and sever the very bonds of human society, those shared interests and shared endeavors that hold together a group of human animals as something qualitatively more than the sum of its parts. In the ancient world, physical distancing *is* social distancing, since all social life takes place in the *agora* and the forum. In the modern, technological world, this is no longer the case. Social institutions and social life may continue to flourish without interruption through the medium of technology. Physical distancing does not necessitate the cessation of social interaction. "Social distancing" is snake oil sold as tonic.

Even taking "social distancing" to mean physical distancing, it is

1 This introduction was composed in late May, 2020.

neither a cure nor a long-term solution, and the most that rational minds hope to gain from self-isolation is a slowing down of the spread of the disease and a postponement of the judgment day. This is not nothing; it buys time for the medical technicians to continue their research, and to hopefully develop an effective treatment or vaccine.

The blind acceptance of "social distancing" as a panacea is the result of ahistorical thinking. This is an idea that no one had ever heard of a few months ago and an idea that would have been news to any great political thinker. It is symptomatic of the widespread faith that our social technicians are invested with an esoteric wisdom of which we know nothing, and which we ought not to question. The vacuity of the term reveals it to be nothing more than a political slogan. Nevertheless, we find ourselves at the mercy of the experts because we are all well aware that we as individuals lack any insight or experience by which to determine for ourselves what is best. We do not know what answer to give to the pressing question, What ought I to do?

Moral philosophy is a contemplation of the good life, or how we ought to live. There is no full human being who has not at some point considered this question. Everyone asks now and again, more or less explicitly, of what the good life consists. "How should I live? Ought I to pursue the contemplative life? the practical life? the life of pleasure?" Very few persons express the questions in so formal a manner, but a calculus of this sort always informs one's endeavors. In normal, everyday situations, experience suggests to us which actions are most likely to yield the results we desire. The experience at work here is nothing profound and philosophical, but the ordinary psychological experience of daily life. The shame of the philosopher is that most human beings, even without a rigorous education in Aristotle, are able to intuit their way toward some semblance of happiness.

It is under extraordinary circumstances that this uncritical instinct for living well breaks down. It is then that we must turn to the wisdom of those who *have* reflected deeply on such crises. For example, in developed nations today, there is a certain level of socio-economic stability on which one may reasonably depend. The doctrine of stoicism, with its imperatives to reflect always upon the fragility of human life and the insignificance of worldly goods, reflects the unstable, violent, and tumultuous world in which men like Zeno and Seneca lived. These conditions are very different from those of the technically regular world of today. Under "normal" circumstances, stoicism is not a useful doctrine. However, under extreme conditions—if one's family is suddenly lost in an accident, or if one is unjustly sentenced to life in prison—the Stoics have a great deal to teach us.

Crises create an imbalance or disconnect between one's worldview and the actual state of the world. When society is turned on its head, new modes of thought and new modes of behavior are needed. Even under the worst conditions, we still seek equilibrium and we recognize the need to consciously reevaluate our ideas about how we ought to live. We can no longer rely on blind instinct, but we lack the tools and knowledge necessary to make informed decisions. Today we confront a global pandemic the likes of which the world has not known for precisely a century. It is safe to say that there are no humans living who can tell us how we ought to comport ourselves. When the living are silent, we must look to the dead.

History does not repeat itself in a tidy manner, but history does evince certain patterns. The same thing does not happen twice, but *kinds* of things happen over and over. The individual's memory has its strict limitations. Fortunately, there is also a collective memory that is infinitely more expansive than that of the individual. You and I have experienced very little, in fact almost nothing. However, the human species has confronted at some time in its enormous past everything beautiful and terrible that wit can imagine. The Ecclesiast says, "What has been is what will be, and what has been done is what will be done; there is nothing new under the sun."[2] When we find ourselves at a loss, confronting something new, we do well to look to our ancestors for guidance. The novel dilemma is prudently confronted with a backward look at the lessons of history. As I have argued elsewhere, progress into the future always involves the recollection of the past.[3]

We have not personally confronted a global pandemic on the scale of COVID-19, but such diseases have regularly tormented the human world in the past. Bubonic plague ravaged both the eastern and western world off and on for nearly fifteen hundred years. The Black Death of 1347-51 killed roughly half of the population of Europe and a third of the population worldwide. This was only one outbreak amongst many. The historian of disease John Kelly writes, "Including the Black Death, three times in recorded human history plague has risen to the level of pandemic.

2 Ecc. 1:9. All Biblical citations refer to *The New Oxford Annotated Bible*, ed. Michael D. Coogan (New York: Oxford, 2001).

3 See my *Memory as Philosophy* (Stuttgart: ibidem, 2019), especially chap. 13 on Hegel's dialectic.

The first time, the Plague of Justinian, is where the story of man and *Y. pestis* begins, and the last time, the Third Pandemic, is where the mysteries of the plague bacillus were finally unraveled."[4] Fatalistic resignation to plague conditions has even informed certain nursery rhymes passed down to us ("Ashes, ashes …"). It is edifying to recall that human beings have suffered worse than us, and yet the species has always managed to survive.

A survey of western literature reveals a large body of classic texts that deal with large-scale medical crises in some respect. This book will subject ten classics to interrogation. Nine of these classics are books from different times and places, written by people with varying proximity to active plague conditions, and the tenth is a film, Ingmar Bergman's *Seventh Seal.* This is more than an idle practice in philosophical meditation; my aim is to extract from each of these works one central lesson that can be applied to the global situation we face today. The great value of recalling the past is its application to present and future problems. The guiding question of this book is, *What can literature teach us about how to live well and prudently during a plague?* This is a question about prudence.

"Prudence" is the name for the classical virtue that applies past wisdom to present dilemmas. In Greek, the word is *phronēsis*, and in Latin *prudentia.* Both terms mean "practical wisdom." Aristotle defines *phronēsis* as "a reasoned and true state of capacity to act with regard to human goods."[5] This is wisdom in acting rightly, as opposed to technē (art), which is wisdom in making. The prudent person is "able to deliberate well about what is good and expedient for himself, not in some particular respect … but about what sorts of things conduce to the good life in general."[6] The good life requires right action, and sound deliberation on right action requires prudence.

The works that I have selected to scrutinize are all great works that bear revisiting time and again. I have limited my selections to texts that are readily available in English, for the benefit of the curious reader who wishes to pursue a complete autodidactic course in plague literature. I have employed no criteria for selection other than my own arbitrary interests. At the end of the text I have included an "Honorable Mention" section that suggests other classic literary works dealing with plagues for the interested reader.

---

4 John Kelly, *The Great Mortality* (New York: HarperCollins, 2005), 41.

5 Aristotle, *Nic. Eth.*, VI.v.1140b20–21. All citations of Aristotle are from *The Complete Works of Aristotle*, 2 vols., ed. Jonathan Barnes (Princeton, NJ: Princeton University Press, 1984).

6 Ibid., VI.v.1140a26–28.

"But surely we modern humans can learn nothing from literary works? A medical problem requires a scientific solution, not an engagement with the humanities. It is technicians that we need." To think in this manner is to reveal one's own limitations. It is the physician's work to treat the body during this pandemic, just as it is the psychologist's work to treat whatever mental health issues arise, and the economist's work to mitigate its economic impact. However, the human being is more than so many pounds of flesh. The human being is a creature with an inner life as well as an epidermis. The question of *how to live well during a pandemic* is not a question for any of these experts, because it is a very different sort of question than how to remain healthy or financially solvent. It is not a technical problem because it concerns acting rather than making. How to live well is a question that can only be hazarded by the humanities, and it can never be satisfactorily resolved in the manner of an equation of physics. If we wish to hear wisdom speaking of matters more spiritual than hand washing and "social distancing," we must turn to the literati.

The "ancient quarrel" between poets and philosophers is much overblown and misunderstood.[7] In its wide, original sense, "poetry" (from *poiesis*, "bringing forth") refers to all artistic creations, not just those rendered into verse. Literature, like philosophy—and like science, religion, technology, and other human practices—aims at understanding the world. No less than these other spheres of knowledge, literature relies upon experience and observation. Where it differentiates itself is in its deliberate use of imagination. The "metaphysics" of poetry is the first wisdom of the world, as Giambattista Vico tells us; it is "not rational and abstract like that of learned men now, but felt imagined as that of those first men who, without power of ratiocination, were all robust sense and vigorous imaginations."[8] The narrative poet's imagination creates situations and characters, and considers how the former affect the latter. Nonetheless, the good poet is still bound by necessity. Certain character types behave in reasonably regular ways under certain conditions. Observation is the proof of this: hubristic men have always tended to do X and are likely to do so in similar circumstances. The narrative poet aims at plausibility. If it is implausible that such a character would behave in such a manner, then the poem is a failure. Obeying the law of plausibility is more important to the poet than

---

7 On the history of this "ancient quarrel," see Raymond Barfield, *The Ancient Quarrel between Philosophy and Poetry* (New York: Cambridge University Press, 2011).

8 Giambattista Vico, *New Science*, trans. Thomas Goddard Bergin and Max Harold Fisch (Ithaca, NY: Cornell University Press, 1988), §375.

obeying the laws of nature. Given what we know about Achilles, it would be strange if in his rage he did *not* fight the river Scamander. Even though this action is impossible, it is still plausible.

The limitation of narrative poetry is its bondage to the concrete. Philosophy begins with the concrete, and moves on to abstractions. Good poetry, however, always conveys more grist for contemplation than meets the eye of a tepid reader. Achilles fighting the river is a scene limited to one particular place and time, but it is also the story of all Achilleses, that is, all humans of Achilles' type. *Finnegans Wake* is the story of all Finnegans (hence the absence of an apostrophe in the title). *Hamlet* is the tragedy of all Hamlets, *Othello* of all Othellos. *The Metamorphosis* is the story of everyone who awakes to find himself transformed into a gigantic bug. It is for this reason that there exists a flourishing academic field known as "philosophy of literature." The imaginative insight of Shakespeare into the character of Hamlet gives the philosopher a starting point or a commonplace for meditation. R. G. Collingwood has justly advised, "The philosopher must go to school with the poets."[9]

Poetic wisdom has much to teach to prudence. Philosophers teach universal ideas, like "the true" and "the good." Scientists teach the nature of the corporeal world. Religious sages teach the relationship between things human and divine. Technicians teach how to fabricate. It is only the poets that teach us how people have lived, felt, behaved, and died under concrete conditions of existence. Poetic truth is not the same as factual truth, but it is equally bound by necessity and is of great interest as an education in living well.

Because, as has already been said, we do not ourselves have any experience in flourishing under plague conditions, it is edifying to look to the concrete works of great poetic minds for guidance. They offer us the key to navigating the unusual pathological conditions that we face today. The characters of *The Betrothed* or *Death in Venice*, much like the character of Achilles, are *not* people radically unlike ourselves, from whom there is no lesson to learn. They are us and we are them. These are books not about particular human individuals, but about all humans who find themselves face to face with plague.

In my meditations upon these classics, I have not bothered to dissect the works in their entirety or to engage with any school of literary

9 R. G. Collingwood, *An Essay on Philosophical Method* (Bristol: Thoemmes, 1995), 214. I use this quotation in a different context than that intended by Collingwood.

criticism. This would be beside the point. Boccaccio's *Decameron* or Thucydides' *Peloponnesian War*, for example, are inexhaustible troves for scholarly books and papers. I do not write this work for scholars, but for anyone and everyone confronting COVID-19 today. It has instead been my intention to use these classic works as a cautious thief treats unearthed treasure chests, stealing a bangle here, a diadem there. I have attempted to abstract from each work one kernel of insight on living well in times of plague, and to crystallize this insight and make clear its relevance to us today. Let us see what our predecessors can teach us in these doubtful and fearsome times. Each chapter focuses on a particular insight I wish to emphasize.

The works considered are discussed in order of publication. These works, in brief overview, are the following:

1. Thucydides' *History of the Peloponnesian War* (c. 400 BCE) describes the Plague of Athens, which caused the deaths of a quarter of all Athenian citizens. The lesson: *pandemics are best confronted by rational, scientific thought, not mythical thought.*
2. Giovanni Boccaccio's *Decameron* (1353) is set during the Black Death, the most deadly catastrophe in history, which took the lives of half of all Europeans. The lesson: *do not abandon the small pleasures of the everyday, and do not lose your sense of humor.*
3. Lorenzo di Filippo Strozzi and Niccolò Machiavelli's *An Epistle Written Concerning the Plague* (1522) narrates a surreal day amidst a fictional Florentine plague. The lesson: *love makes pandemics more bearable, and romance can still be kindled even during an outbreak.*
4. François Rabelais' *Gargantua and Pantagruel* (1532-64) contains reflections on bubonic plague from a trained and practicing physician. The lesson: *the plague is not divine punishment, and superstitious behavior expedites the damage.*
5. Daniel Defoe's *A Journal of the Plague Year* (1722) was written to remind the people of England of the horrors of the 1665 Great Plague of London. The lesson: *plague conditions require a disciplined quarantine maintained by wisdom, not compulsion.*
6. Alessandro Manzoni's *The Betrothed* (1827) is partly set during the 1630 plague of Milan, which violently upends the situation of the characters of the story. The lesson: *crises disrupt the course of life, and present an opportunity for forgiveness and the reorganization of passions.*

7. Thomas Mann's *Death in Venice* (1912) takes place in Venice during a cholera epidemic that becomes increasingly invasive. The lesson: *do not allow the Dionysian impulses to gain the upper hand*, or, *restrain the passionate element of life*.
8. Albert Camus' *The Plague* (1947) narrates the struggles of the population of Oran, Algeria during a fictional outbreak of plague in the 1940s. The lesson: *practice common decency*.
9. Ingmar Bergman's *The Seventh Seal* (1957) follows a handful of characters trying to evade Death and survive the Black Death in Sweden. The lesson: *the charitable deed in times of despair redeems the world.*
10. José Saramago's *Blindness* (1995) portrays the fate of the people of an unnamed country that is plagued with an outbreak of a fictional disease that causes white blindness. The lesson: *in order to flourish during pandemics, it is imperative that communities work together.*

All of these are excellent poetic works in their own right, as accessible in times of robust health as in times of plague. They have much to teach us when we are well, but we find other lessons when we read them under the auspices of our own pandemic.

In general, these crises have all been referred to as "plagues," whether this title is strictly appropriate or not. The term "pandemic" does not have a long history. The *Oxford English Dictionary* dates its first use as an adjective to Gideon Harvey's *Morbus Anglicus* of 1666, and its first use as a noun to 1846. In Greek, the term means "all the people." It refers to a disease with outbreaks in all or most regions of the world, as opposed to an epidemic, which is more regional in nature. "Plague" today refers to a specific infectious disease caused by the bacterium identified as *Yersinia pestis*, and sub-classified into different strains. However, the causes and mode of transmission of plague were unknown to epidemiology until 1894. In literature prior to this time, the term "plague" is a general, informal term for any medical pandemic. In the title for this book, I have used the term "plague" in its informal sense, in place of the word "pandemic," so as to confront the works of literature I wish to discuss on their own terms.

We have all had to become doctors, now that the world is characterized by disease. How do we do this? In the *Republic* of Plato, Socrates suggests, "The cleverest doctors are those who, in addition to learning their craft, have had contact with the greatest number of very sick bodies from childhood on, have themselves experienced every illness, and aren't very healthy by nature."[10] Much familiarity with disease is a necessary education for anyone who would hope to overcome disease. Ought we to make ourselves ill? to pursue exotic pathologies for the sake of the experience? Certainly not. However, we can do so vicariously through a close engagement with the literature of disease. We can come to know our enemy, and come to know what strategies others have used when confronting such an enemy. In knowing what others have done, we gain self-knowledge, for all humans partake equally of what Montaigne called "the human condition." We equip ourselves with the wisdom of experience and we turn ourselves into doctors intimately familiar with the malady. This is wisdom of the soul, which is the guide of the body.

If we are able to learn from the poets and to internalize their insights, then we will understand what prudence demands of us today. We will have a sense of what moral philosophy demands, that is, how we ought to live and how we ought to think about ourselves and our relationship to others and to society as a whole under these unusual conditions. This work is an education in equilibrium. The return to the poets is an effort to find a rule for behavior in a time when all of the social rules we uncritically accept have been compromised or overturned. The poets offer hope for discovering a firm footing, a *topos*, during this crisis. This is surely better medicine than the hollow slogan "social distancing."

For the first edition of this book, thanks are due to: David N. Bahr, Megan Lillie, Gregory A. McBrayer, Zuzana Vanha Montagne, Erin Peone, Rolland G. Smith, and Donald Phillip Verene. For the second edition: Jehanne Gheith, Alexander L. Gungov, Friedrich C. Luft, Brian P. Quaranta, the Trent Center for Bioethics, Humanities, and History of Medicine at Duke University, and the editorial personnel at ibidem.

10 Plato, *Rep.* III, 408d–e. All references to Plato are from *Complete Works*, ed. John M. Cooper (Indianapolis: Hackett, 1997).

CHAPTER I

Thucydides

The Peloponnesian War

Think Rationally, Not Mythically

The Peloponnesian War (431–404 BCE), fought primarily between factions led by Athens and Sparta, was one of the epochal events of ancient Europe. It engulfed the whole of the world known at the time to the Greeks, and its massive extent compelled the establishment of new political modes and institutions that had a significant influence on the direction of all subsequent European history. The Peloponnesian War is an event from the past that is never fully past, and its lessons are rediscovered by every generation. The great chronicler of this war was Thucydides of Athens (c. 460–400 BCE), one of the pioneers of the evidence-based historical method. Thucydides was a first-hand witness to much of the war as a combatant. He wrote his History of the Peloponnesian War "in the belief that it was going to be a great war and more worth writing about than any of those which had taken place in the past" (I.1).[1]

In 430 BCE, the second year of the war, Athens was struck by the outbreak of a pernicious epidemic. This epidemic was referred to as the Plague of Athens, "plague" being used in its general sense. The exact pathology of the disease is not clear, and modern researchers have posited smallpox and typhus as possible diagnoses.[2] The plague was devastating, resulting in as many as 100,000 Athenian deaths (roughly a quarter of the population of the city at the time). Athens did not sufficiently recover to mount a major offensive attack for over a decade, and this misfortune ultimately played a decisive role in the outcome of the war and the future balance of power in Greece. Thucydides' account is the only firsthand description of the epidemic that has survived.

This plague was particularly excruciating for its victims. Thucydides writes, "People in perfect health suddenly began to have burning feelings in the head; their eyes became red and inflamed; inside their mouths there

1 Parenthetical citations in this section refer to Thucydides, *History of the Peloponnesian War*, trans. Rex Warner (New York: Penguin, 1985), by book and paragraph numbers.

2 See Robert J. Littman, "The Plague of Athens: Epidemiology and Paleopathology," *Mount Sinai Journal of Medicine* 76 (2009): 456–67.

was bleeding from the throat and tongue, and the breath became unnatural and unpleasant." This was followed by respiratory symptoms and "vomiting of every kind of bile that has been given a name by the medical profession," as well as "small pustules and ulcers." Many victims died seven or eight days from the onset of symptoms from "internal fever." For survivors of this critical period, the disease "descended to the bowels, producing violent ulceration and uncontrollable diarrhea, so that most of them died later as a result of the weakness caused by this." In other cases, it affected "the genitals, the fingers, and the toes, and many of those who recovered lost the use of these members; some, too, went blind. There were some also who, when they first began to get better, suffered from a total loss of memory" (II.49). Thucydides bore witness to his neighbors dying in this manner all about him, and contracted the disease himself at one point (II.48). He laments, "Words indeed fail one when one tries to give a general picture of this disease; and as for the sufferings of individuals, they seemed almost beyond the capacity of individuals to endure" (II.50).

On what can such visible suffering be blamed by persons prone to look for meaning in events? There is a marked tendency amongst the ancient pagans to associate misfortune with the anger of the gods (and we will see when discussing Rabelais that monotheistic religions sometimes share this tendency). When Homer's Iliad begins, the Greek camp is beset by an outbreak of plague. Homer tells us that Apollo, angered by Agamemnon's impiety in abducting Chryseis, the daughter of his priest, has sent this devastating plague to chastise the Greek soldiers: "Incensed at the king / he swept a fatal plague through the army—men were dying."[3] The plague only abates when Odysseus returns Chryseis to her father, thereby appeasing the wrath of Apollo. The tragedy of Sophocles' Oedipus Rex is set in motion by Oedipus' ill-fated efforts to appease the gods in order to end a plague with which they ravage Thebes. The Delphic oracle tells the Thebans that the plague is a divine punishment for the iniquity of the Thebans in allowing a regicide to go unpunished. Only by driving the criminal from the land will Thebes be relieved from this epidemic: "King Phoebus in plain words commanded us / to drive out a pollution from our land."[4] The horrors of the plague are emphasized even more strongly in Seneca's retelling of the story:

> The killing plague; death pays no heed to age

3 Homer, *The Iliad*, trans. Robert Fagles (New York: Penguin, 1998), Bk. I, lines 10–11.

4 Sophocles, *Oedipus the King*, in *Sophocles I*, trans. David Grene, ed. D. Grene and Richmond Lattimore (Chicago: University of Chicago Press, 1991), lines 97–98.

> Or sex; young men and old, fathers and sons—
> The mortal pestilence makes no distinction.
> Husband and wife await one funeral pyre,
> And there are no more tears to mourn the dead.[5]

In Rome, Fever (Febris) was a significant enough matter of concern to be elevated to the level of a goddess, and votaries would pray at her altars in order to keep disease at bay. Cicero was critical of this worship: "So far did this sort of error go, that even harmful things were not only given the names of gods but actually had forms of worship instituted in their honour: witness the temple to Fever on the Palatine. ... Let us therefore banish from philosophy entirely the error of making assertions in discussing the immortal gods that are derogatory to their dignity."[6] However, Cicero was an outlier. The cult flourished enough for Rome to support three temples dedicated to Febris, the principle one on the Palatine. Across the ancient pagan world, it was a commonplace that pandemics were divine punishment for the iniquity of mortals, and could only be kept at bay by supplication and sacrifice.

Thucydides recognizes and acknowledges this popular opinion about the origin of contagion. At times he even "invites" his readers to think of the plague and the other disasters suffered by the Athenians as "destined punishments for its insolence and injustice,"[7] though he never endorses this view. Thucydides writes, "Old stories of past prodigies, which had not found much confirmation in recent experience, now became credible. Wide areas, for instance, were affected by violent earthquakes; there were more frequent eclipses of the sun than had ever been recorded before; in various parts of the country there were extensive droughts followed by famine; and there was the plague which did more harm and destroyed more life than almost any other single factor. All these calamities fell together upon the Hellenes after the outbreak of the war" (I.23). In the absence of natural explanations, it is understandable that this panoply of evils would be interpreted in light of old prophecies and prodigies. However, there are better interpretations.

For his time, Thucydides is a rare rationalist who looks for the natural causes rather than the divine causes of calamities. The plague

5 Lucius Annaeus Seneca, *Oedipus*, in *Four Tragedies and Octavia*, trans. E. F. Watling (Baltimore: Penguin, 1974), lines 46–50.

6 Marcus Tullius Cicero, *De natura Deorum*, trans. H. Rackham (Cambridge, MA: Harvard University Press, 1979), III.xxv.63–64.

7 David Bolotin, "Thucydides," in *History of Political Philosophy*, ed. Leo Strauss and Joseph Cropsey (Chicago: University of Chicago Press, 1987), 15.

disproportionately struck Athens, but it was not limited to Athens alone, nor did it begin in Europe. Thucydides writes, "The plague originated, so they say, in Ethiopia in upper Egypt, and spread from there into Egypt itself and Libya and much of the territory of the king of Persia. In the city of Athens it appeared suddenly, and the first cases were among the population of Piraeus" (II.48). Piraeus was Athens' only commercial port. The implication is that contagion began in northern Africa and western Asia and crossed the Mediterranean Sea on trading vessels. The fact that the disease affected multiple kingdoms and arrived relatively late at Athens suggests to unprejudiced human reason that the plague was not a supernatural chastisement sent directly from the gods unto the Athenians. There is no celestial "meaning" behind its outbreak, no *mysterium* for the oracles and priests to decipher. Its spread is the result of the intermingling of peoples brought together by commercial interests, and the disease passes from human to human rather from divine to human. Because Thucydides is not a physician, he does not speculate on the origin of pathogens: "As to the question of how it could first have come about or what causes can be found adequate to explain its powerful effect on nature, I must leave that to be considered by other writers, with or without medical experience" (II.48). He leaves no doubt, however, that there are such causes and conditions, and that the epidemic can be explained without recourse to offended divinity.

Thucydides' position grounds the plague in *phusis*, nature, rather than *meta ta phusika*, metaphysics. All of his observations, based on empirical evidence, argue against investing the plague with religious or mythical significance. He stops short of explicitly denying divine intervention, but his suggestions have the compulsory power of demonstrations. The reader of Thucydides cannot doubt that the gods were absent while Athens suffered. He writes that "prayers made in the temples, consultation of oracles, and so forth" were of no use in meliorating the effects of the plague (II.47). Nor did piety have any connection to survival: "As for the gods, it seemed to be the same thing whether one worshipped them or not, when one saw the good and the bad dying indiscriminately" (II.53). Taking sanctuary at the sacred altars availed nothing, and temples "were full of the dead bodies of people who had died inside them" (II.52). Thucydides goes so far as to ridicule the superstitious Greek reliance on the oracles. An old oracle was recalled that said, "War with the Dorians comes, and a death will come at the same time." However, it had been unclear at the time whether the oracle had said "death" or "dearth." Thucydides writes, "In the present state of affairs the view that the word was 'death' naturally prevailed; it was a case of people adapting their memories to suit their sufferings. Certainly I think that if there is ever another war with the Dorians after this one, and if a dearth results from it, then in all probability people will quote the other version" (II.54). No other ancient writer would dare to handle the oracles with such glibness until Cicero.

For Thucydides, blaming Athenian arrogance for calling cosmic wrath upon itself is counter-productive. If the gods will have blood, there is nothing left for human endeavor to undertake. It is beyond the power of human beings to defy what the Olympians and the *Moirai* (Fates) have set in motion. The psychological consequence of resigning oneself to the belief in divine chastisement is hopeless fatalism and a crisis of self-confidence. Thucydides suggests that this dogmatism is actively harmful. He says that of all the horrors of the epidemic, "The most terrible thing of all was the despair into which people fell when they realized that they had caught the plague; for they would immediately adopt an attitude of utter hopelessness, and, by giving in in this way, would lose their powers of resistance" (II.51). The psychological despair of believing oneself to be out of favor with the gods becomes an aggravating circumstance of the epidemic. We will encounter several other pernicious consequences of this belief in the work of later writers.

The disfavor of the gods is particularly devastating to the Athenian people given the context of the plague within Thucydides' *History*. In the text, the scene in which the plague strikes immediately follows the famous public funeral oration given by Pericles, then ruler of Athens (though the two events were separated by several months in historical time). In this oration, Pericles honors those who lost their lives in the first year of the war, praises the greatness of Athens, and praises in particular its military acumen: "Athens, alone of the states we know, comes to her testing time in a greatness that surpasses what was imagined of her. In her case, and in her case alone, no invading enemy is ashamed at being defeated, and no subject can complain of being governed by people unfit for their responsibilities. Mighty indeed are the marks and monuments of our empire which we have left" (II.41). Pericles exhorts the people of Athens to live up to the greatness of the dead. This oration is a high point for the Athenians, in which their glory and might is extolled. Their confidence is at its height, and they fully believe in their own prowess as soldiers, the political and military aptitude of their governors, and the favor of fortune. The plague interrupts this state of affairs and plunges Athens at once into one of its lowest and darkest points in the narrative.

Such a rapid reversal of fortunes is psychologically disorienting. Athenian greatness was so obvious as to be taken as a premise for oratorical demonstrations. Pericles says, "What I would prefer is that you should fix your eyes every day on the greatness of Athens as she really is, and should fall in love with her" (II.43). His exhortation could be framed, "Because Athens is great, if we Athenians live up to the standards of our forebears, we must succeed in battle." Athenian exceptionalism was foundational knowledge for the people of the city. Foundational knowledge, like language, is a part of the basic conceptual system by which human beings acquire knowledge about particular things. The greatness of Athens was a certainty that was the ground of many other beliefs and aspirations. The plague was the most significant humiliation the city had faced up to that time, and it undermined the extreme self-confidence that was embedded in the average Athenian psyche. When foundational knowledge is falsified, the psyche becomes disoriented and many secondary structures of belief crumble. The subject's entire worldview is shaken, and he or she tries to make sense of the unexpected blow. In wretched desperation, the beleaguered people lament with the Psalmist, "My God, my God, why have you forsaken me?"[8]

History shows that most sociable behavior is rooted in the need to impose order on nature and to mitigate its many unpredictable dangers. Knowledge and reason are the characteristically human instruments that allow us to contend against a chaotic world and to establish a level of tranquility. Under ordinary conditions, human beings uncritically invest certain individuals and institutions with authority over certain spheres. These are the individuals who have most rigorously studied the field, mastered its methods and techniques, and demonstrated an aptitude for using this knowledge to bring about preferable outcomes. Generals are handed control of military maneuvers, pundits are trusted for political analysis, and the financial forecasts of economists shape market behavior. These people are seen as masters of the rationality particular to their respective fields. However, unexpected catastrophes compromise this public faith. The catastrophe appears to be evidence that reason, even at its highest level, is insufficient to ensure order and tranquility. When reason fails to answer the urgent needs of the group, the masses are faced with a crisis of confidence. The tendency of human beings at such times is to lose faith in reason, and to revert to other modes of thought in hopes of salvation. The

8 Ps. 22:1.

most significant lesson taught by Thucydides is that *pandemics are best confronted by rational, scientific thought, not mythical thought.*

The philosopher Ernst Cassirer referred to the myriad modes of thinking as "symbolic forms." Rational or scientific thinking is one such form, which is usually dominant in the modern world, but it is always possible to adopt other forms of thought. Art, religion, language, and myth are among the symbolic forms that tend to precede rational thinking in the history of the human species. These forms are not just hermeneutical; they actively *produce* the human world. Cassirer writes, "Myth, art, language and science appear as symbols; not in the sense of mere figures which refer to some given reality by means of suggestion and allegorical renderings, but in the sense of forces each of which produces and posits a world of its own. … Thus the special symbolic forms are not imitations, but *organs* of reality, since it is solely by their agency that anything real becomes an object for intellectual apprehension, and as such is made visible to us."[9] There is no world except a meaningful world, and meaning is produced through the operation of symbolic forms. The modern human being with some understanding of meteorology sees a lightning storm as the effect of negatively and positively charged particles, but our ancestors literally beheld the wrath of Jove. Both apprehensions are simply true.

The symbolic forms of cognition do not absorb or replace one another as consciousness comes to maturity. Science is not, as is sometimes said, enlightened mythology. The rational, scientific consciousness that dominates the contemporary world is only one mode of thought among others, not the completion of a series. For Cassirer, the various symbolic forms are autonomous, each governed by its own laws. All of them coexist in human consciousness at any stage of development as possible modes of thought. He writes, "Each form, in a manner of speaking, is assigned to a special plane, within which it fulfills itself and develops its specific character in total independence."[10] One form or another is dominant at a particular moment, but it cannot annihilate the others. Abandoned symbolic forms become the background of thought, and retain the potential for recrudescence. Mythical thinking always haunts rational thinking, and however "enlightened" and scientifically advanced the society may be, a general reversion to mythical thinking is always possible. This

9 Ernst Cassirer, *Language and Myth*, trans. Susanne K. Langer (New York: Dover, 1946), 8.

10 Cassirer, *The Philosophy of Symbolic Forms*, trans. Ralph Manheim (New Haven, CT: Yale University Press, 1955), I:95.

becomes much more likely when the violence of the world requires immediate action and the efficacy of reason is in doubt. Crises like the plague and the later military disasters suffered by the Athenians open the door to such conditions. The cultured men and women of the Age of Pericles become timorous and superstitious troglodytes at the first report of plague.

What does it mean to think mythically rather than rationally? Cassirer refers to the function of the mythical form of consciousness as the "expressive function." In mythical thinking, this expressive function is inseparable from the immediacy of perception. For Cassirer, myth is perception itself as a way of thinking. He writes, "There is so little conflict between the content of perception and the form of myth that the two grow together and fuse into a thoroughly concrete unity."[11] Religion thereby produces the very character of the world through expression. There is a logic at play, but one in which there are no fixed identities or classes of objects; the logic of myth is similar to the logic of dreams. To pre-rational perception, particular things are always *sui generis*. They belong to no "classes" or "types," and the rules by which they behave are particular to themselves alone. There is no such thing as a universal law. Each thing possesses its own unique demon: this apple does not fall to the ground because all apples fall, but because the demon in this particular apple so desires. Even the identity of the same thing is not fixed through time. When the shaman puts on the mask and becomes the God, he literally *becomes* the God. Symbolic meaning is pregnant in everything and expresses itself immediately to the perceiving subject, bypassing the mediation of reflection. The basic categories in which things express themselves are as benign or malignant.

It would be impossible for any culture to survive if its thinking was *entirely* mythical. Human existence depends on the recognition of at least some basic universals. One kind of thing gives sustenance to the body, and another is harmful; one time of year is right for sewing the fields, and another for harvesting the crops. However, there have been many human groups that have flourished with a framework of thinking that is mostly mythical.

During the long Age of Pericles that had preceded the plague, Athens was remarkable among the Greek city-states for its rationality, cultivation of science and the arts, and good civic order. Nevertheless, we see from Thucydides' narrative that when the Athenians suffered the calamity of the plague, many of them quickly fell into a mythical mode of thinking. The Periclean government at first adopted rational measures to try to mitigate

---

11 Ibid., III:61.

the damage of the epidemic, ordering the removal of people from the countries to the cities and establishing mass graves for the dead, though these maneuvers only served to aggravate the damage of the plague (II.52). No means of preservation was effective, and no rule of the spread of contagion was apparent. People in perfect health were struck down with the sudden onset of the disease. The plague ravaged in the manner of the gods, indiscriminately and without rhyme or reason. It became readily apparent that the plague was beyond the power of rationality to address. The result was the rapid disintegration of lawful civic order.

Thucydides writes, "The catastrophe was so overwhelming that men, not knowing what would happen next to them, became indifferent to every rule of religion or of law" (II.52). Athens descended into "the beginnings of a state of unprecedented lawlessness. Seeing how quick and abrupt were the changes of fortune which came to the rich who suddenly died and to those who had previously been penniless but now inherited their wealth, people now began openly to venture on acts of self-indulgence which before then they used to keep dark. Thus they resolved to spend their money quickly and to spend it on pleasure, since money and life seemed equally ephemeral." The rules and norms that had governed social and economic behavior lost their compulsory power. The immediacy of pleasure expressed itself as a higher value than any of the abstract goods that require reflection on universals. Thucydides continues, "As for what is called honour, no one showed himself willing to abide by its laws, so doubtful was it whether one would survive to enjoy the name for it. It was generally agreed that what was both honourable and valuable was the pleasure of the moment. … As for offences against human law, no one expected to live long enough to be brought to trial and punished" (II.53).

All of the practices that bind human beings together in society assume a shared faith in a relatively stable and predictable future. This presupposes the capacity of reason to discover universal rules of cause and effect. Humans are obedient to law because they believe its enforcement ensures a more orderly state of affairs in general. They save and invest money because they are confident in market stability. Both practices accept universal norms. The Athenians under plague conditions lost their faith in general rules. They became lawless as soon as nature ceased to behave rationally. Immediate pleasure came to supersede long-term stability as the highest good. Human action was no longer mediated by reflection. When this happens, self-control is altogether sacrificed. Where there is no self-control, no rule for living well beyond the moment, and no thought beyond immediate perception, we have a society that has abandoned reason and adopted a mythical attitude toward the world. "Utter hopelessness" (II.59) turns humans away from authorities and statesmen. The only guidance they admit is the auspices of the birds and the thunder. The particulars of the world express themselves immediately as malignant or benign, and this expression determines individual behavior.

The harm done by the embrace of mythical thinking is evident. Coordinated group action becomes impossible. Men and women turn away from orderliness and descend into self-indulgent hedonism. Despair of human efficacy produces either a pernicious nihilism or a quaking before the divine,[12] and both positions render the individual socially useless. Without self-control, there can be no science, no arts, and no culture whatsoever. Where humans exist but have forsaken culture, there is only barbarism. Groups that think mythically are not governed by law, but by custom, and custom arises from the objects of nature expressing themselves to perception. Plague is a thunderbolt from the gods. If the gods are chastising Athens, then it is the end of civilization, and all things become permissible. Mythical thinking in itself is neither good nor bad, but when it erupts within societies that are already developed, it tends to have a rapid regressive effect. This opens an entire Pandora's box of evils, letting loose all manner of "sad troubles for mankind."[13]

What was true for the ancient Greeks remains true today, and thus the counsel of Thucydides remains pertinent. Mythical thinking is not a phenomenon foreign to us. It is modern arrogance to believe that ours is a world immune to myth. In the words of Georges Bataille, "The absence of myth is also a myth: the coldest, the purest, the only *true* myth."[14] Crises both real and apparent continue to undermine our faith in reason and lead to mythical modes of understanding the world. Economic, military, and medical disasters all throw people back upon mythical tribalism. To remain reasonable in a world gone wrong requires constant vigilance.

Cassirer demonstrated in *The Myth of the State* that the rise of German National Socialism in the first half of the twentieth century was rooted in this phenomenon. Nazi ideology arose at a time when Germans, much

12 Giambattista Vico uses the term *spavento*, utter terror, to refer to the trembling felt by man when he feels himself under the gaze of Jove the Thunderer. See *New Science*, §502.

13 Hesiod, *Works and Days*, trans. Richmond Lattimore (Ann Arbor, MI: University of Michigan Press, 1991), line 95.

14 Georges Bataille, *The Absence of Myth*, trans. Michael Richardson (New York: Verso, 1994), 48.

like the Athenians, faced shattered self-confidence and debilitating socio-economic conditions. This instability shook the faith of many Germans in reason and intellectual authority. The leaders of the Nazi party exploited this crisis and developed a technique of political myth. Cassirer writes, "Myth has always been described as the result of an unconscious activity and as a free product of imagination. But here we find myth made according to plan. The new political myths do not grow up freely. … They are artificial things fabricated by very skillful and cunning artisans. It has been reserved for the twentieth century, our own great technical age, to develop a new technique of myth."[15] The first step in this fabrication of myth is transforming the function of language, replacing descriptive or semantic words with emotive, "magical" words. The second step is the introduction of new special rituals that distinguish "us" from "them". Finally, the leader takes on the qualities of "*homo magus*" and "*homo divinans*," both prophet and savior.[16]

Political myth remains prominent today. We find that the political language of America is primarily emotive ("Obamacare," "Crooked Hillary," etc.); rites with little history serve to distinguish cultural groups (standing or kneeling for the national anthem at sporting events); and we respond to the leaders of our nation as tribal culture heroes, either benevolent or malicious, rather than as human beings (this is equally true of Barack Obama and Donald Trump). We are as susceptible to mythical thinking as every other civilization throughout history.

The lesson to be learned from Thucydides is that we must resist the urge to view pandemics as divine chastisement, and we must preserve our faith in reason even when it fails and mythical modes of thought seem more edifying. The world health community, and in particular the American public health institutions, have failed to enact sufficient preventative measures. The political and economic leaders of America have likewise failed to implement timely or decisive policies for maintaining good order. Different institutions and authorities blame one another for these failures, but in truth, none has demonstrated due foresight or prudence. The complex systems established by technical reason to preserve the status quo have proven themselves ineffective, and each week reveals further defects in these systems. It is easy in such circumstances to lose faith in reason altogether. It is easy to abandon one's calling, abandon one's duties, and embrace a hedonistic or superstitious worldview.

---

15 Cassirer, *The Myth of the State* (New Haven, CT: Yale University Press, 1973), 282.

16 Ibid., 282–89.

This is a temptation that we must work to avoid. The result would be a loss of self-control, and a consequent breakdown of public order. A breakdown of this type has threatened America since the inception of shelter in place orders. Passionate, uncritical outrage (born of the sense of impotence and abandonment) has yielded nation-wide protests against these orders and reckless behavior amongst malcontents. Thucydides depicted the aggravating chaos resulting from thinking mythically during a pandemic. Prudence demands that we internalize this lesson from the Athenians. By no means is rationality an absolute guarantee of security. It has misfired many times in the past and will continue to do so in the future. Mythical solutions can often be the best means of confronting minor problems. However, experience has shown that global disasters can only be mitigated by rational thinking. Acting rightly in crisis situations requires rehabilitating and correcting reason, not abandoning it. To abandon reason at such times and to act on unrestrained passion is to compound a medical crisis with social anarchy.

CHAPTER II

Giovanni Boccaccio

The Decameron

Keep Your Sense of Humor

The Black Death was the most deadly disaster in the history of the world. Over a six year period (1347–53), this severe strain of bubonic plague indiscriminately ravaged all nations. It was responsible for the death of between fifty and two hundred million people worldwide, including roughly half the population of Europe. It is thought to have been carried from Asia to Europe aboard Genoese trade ships, and to have first appeared in Sicily, later spreading through mainland Italy to the rest of the continent. Italy's position at the epicenter of this pandemic is attributable to its role as the center of Mediterranean trade. The Black Death marked the start of what is now called the Second Plague Pandemic, which continued to flare up in Europe until the middle of the eighteenth century.[1] The effects of this catastrophe on European psychology and culture were enormous and reached into all aspects of human life.

A particularly devastating outbreak occurred in Florence in 1348, between the months of March and July. Niccolò Machiavelli says that "more than ninety-six thousand souls in Florence were lost" in that time.[2] All told, between one half and two thirds of the city's population perished in those four months.[3] It would be centuries before the population of the city would return to what it had been prior to 1348. The best firsthand description of the Florentine outbreak was written by Giovanni Boccaccio (1313–75), the first Italian master of prose, in the introduction to the first day of his *Decameron*, which was conceived, written, and published while the Black Death was active.

The *Decameron* (Greek for "ten days") is structured as a series of vignettes (*novelle*) told by ten characters over the course of two weeks.

---

1 See Frank M. Snowden, *Epidemics and Society* (New Haven, CT: Yale University Press, 2020), 36–38.

2 Niccolò Machiavelli, *Florentine Histories*, trans. Laura F. Banfield and Harvey C. Mansfield, Jr. (Princeton, NJ: Princeton University Press, 1988), 104.

3 John M. Najemy, *A History of Florence, 1200—1575* (Malden, MA: Blackwell, 2008), 97. Other estimates, notably Samuel K. Cohn's, suggest that as much as four fifths of the city's population died of plague.

The group does not engage in this entertainment on holy days or on one day a week designated for chores, making ten total evenings in which stories are told. These vignettes are united by a frame story in a manner similar to Geoffrey Chaucer's *Canterbury Tales* or the *Arabian Nights*. The frame story is set during the outbreak of the plague in Florence. The group of young Florentines—seven women and three men—flee from the city to a villa in Fiesole in order to avoid infection. Their storytelling is a means of passing the time and distracting themselves from the horrors around them. The stories range from didactic moral tales to stories of erotic love to Boccaccio's specialty, ribald and scandalous tales of human folly.

The frame story begins by describing the horrors of the plague, as well as characterizing the attitude of Florentines towards the pandemic. To introduce the situation in Florence, Boccaccio writes, "The sum of thirteen hundred and forty-eight years had elapsed since the fruitful Incarnation of the Son of God, when the noble city of Florence, which for its great beauty excels all others in Italy, was visited by the deadly pestilence. Some say that it descended upon the human race through the influence of the heavenly bodies, others that it was a punishment signifying God's righteous anger at our iniquitous way of life. ... In the face of its onrush, all the wisdom and ingenuity of man were unavailing" (50).[4] He then begins a description of the progress of the plague in its victims: "Its earliest appearance, in men and women alike, was the appearance of certain swellings in the groin or the armpit. ... Later on, the symptoms of the disease changed, and many people began to find dark blotches and bruises on their arms, thighs, and other parts of the body." Once these signs were observed, few people recovered, and "in most cases death occurred within three days from the appearance of the symptoms we have described, some people dying more rapidly than others" (50–51).

Boccaccio admits that his narrative about the plague is "a remarkable story," one that "were it not for the fact that I am one of many people who saw it with their own eyes, I would scarcely dare to believe it, let alone commit it to paper" (51). This story includes otherwise sound men falling ill and dying in a matter of days, and sometimes falling dead on the spot; parents refusing to care for children, lovers for beloved, and many dying alone without aid who might have been saved; corpses lying in piles on the streets or rotting unattended inside homes; enormous trenches dug and filled with anonymous bodies; the fringe elements of society engaging in

4 All parenthetical citations in this section refer to Giovanni Boccaccio, *The Decameron*, trans. G. H. McWilliam (New York: Penguin, 1972).

open lawlessness (51–57). The proximity of death and the grip of terror brought about a widespread loss of respect for the victims of the outbreak: "There were no tears or candles or mourners to honour the dead; in fact, no more respect was accorded to dead people than would nowadays be shown towards dead goats" (56). Boccaccio laments that in the spring of 1348 alone "it is reliably thought that over a hundred thousand human lives were extinguished within the walls of the city of Florence. Yet before this lethal catastrophe fell upon the city, it is doubtful whether anyone would have guessed it contained so many inhabitants" (57–58). In a few months' time, the vast majority of the city's population was dead, the fatal pestilence striking swiftly and often without warning, and both noble and common households were reduced to nothing.

Boccaccio observes that many Florentines held the opinion that "there was no better or more efficacious remedy against a plague than to run away from it" (53). We will see that Daniel Defoe believes that flight is the best method of self-preservation during a local epidemic. However, such a strategy is much less effective when the outbreak is global. Boccaccio says that though flight may be the safest of all courses of action, it is still not terribly effective. Not all of those who fled Florence in the year of the plague died, but by no means did all survive.

Lacking a better alternative, the young women in the frame story of the *Decameron* make up their minds to flee the city—which promises certain death—and to hazard their fates in remote isolation. In the fourteenth century, venturing outside one's city walls was rare, but such actions become obligatory when to remain is to bear witness every day to the complete disintegration of all marks of civilization. The eldest of the young women counsels, "Here we linger for no other purpose, or so it seems to me, than to count the number of corpses being taken to burial. ... And if we go outside, we shall see the dead and the sick being carried hither and thither" (59).

Florence in 1348 was a gallery of horrors, a city of the dead and for the dead. It was T. S. Eliot's wasteland,

> Unreal city,
> Under the brown fog of a winter dawn,
> A crowd flowed over London Bridge, so many,
> I had not thought death had undone so many.[5]

The bloated corpses lining the streets far outnumbered the living. Like war,

5 T. S. Eliot, "The Wasteland," in *The Complete Plays and Poems: 1909–1950* (New York: Harcourt, Brace & World, 1962), lines 60–63.

plague nullifies entire social networks overnight and socially orphans those who do not perish. Survivors are left without orientation and without hope. The story-tellers of the *Decameron* have seen friends and family struck down in the bloom of health, heard the groans of parents and siblings falling ill and rapidly perishing in the next room. They have despaired of their own survival. The pathetic lot of the survivor is captured by Boccaccio's young woman: "My house was once full of servants, and now that there is no one left apart from my maid and myself, I am filled with foreboding and feel as if every hair of my head is standing on end. Wherever I go in the house, wherever I pause to rest, I seem to be haunted by the shades of the departed, whose faces no longer appear as I remember them but with strange and horribly twisted expressions that frighten me out of my senses" (60). The women are compelled to invite three young male companions to accompany them on their retreat because "our own menfolk are dead, and those few that are still alive are fleeing in scattered little groups from that which we too are intent upon avoiding" (62).

What does the decade of refugees hope to gain from this flight and isolation? Pleasure is the object, but not the dissolute carnal pleasure into which so many Florentines had descended. Despite Boccaccio's reputation as a writer of immoral tales, he is never an advocate of immoralism. One reason the group leaves Florence is to avoid the nihilistic hedonism erupting amongst the living. Rather than vulgar pleasure, the storytellers seek the pleasures of beauty and nature, pure air, brisk exercise, and good cheer. The eldest woman counsels, "We could go and stay together on one of our various country estates, shunning at all costs the lewd practices of our fellow citizens and feasting and merrymaking as best we may without in any way overstepping the bounds of what is reasonable. There we shall hear the birds singing, we shall see fresh green hills and plains, fields of corn undulating like the sea, and trees of at least a thousand different species; and we shall have a clearer view of the heavens, which, troubled though they are, do not however deny us their eternal beauties" (61). When the group reaches the abandoned villa, they are gratified by such simple pleasures as "delectable gardens and meadows," "wells of cool, refreshing water," and cellars "stocked with precious wines" (64).

The plague is an external enemy, beyond the control of the individual. These simple pleasures, though, remain in the power of individuals, and cannot be alienated by any foreign evil. However wretched the world becomes, it remains within the power of the human spirit to live well, to appreciate beauty, and to remain upright. Disease can end one's life, but has no power over the delectability of life unless the subject grants it that power. This view of the situation is implicit in the behavior of the young men and women of the *Decameron*'s frame story. Such a view is characteristic of the ancient Stoic philosophers, and owes much to their influence. From Epictetus we learn to ask the questions, "I must die. But must I die bawling? I must be put in chains—but moaning and groaning too? I must be exiled; but is there anything to keep me from going with a smile, calm and self-composed?"[6] Seneca counsels, "Nothing bad *can* happen to a good man. ... Adversity's onslaughts are powerless to affect the spirit of a brave man: it remains unshaken and makes all events assume its own colour; for it is stronger than all external forces."[7] In the case of personal tragedy, grief and despair must be restrained and must not compromise one's composure, "for even in expressing grief there is such a thing as moderation."[8]

Boccaccio represents this stoical attitude as the most edifying position to take amidst nightmarish conditions. There is nothing one can do to raise the dead or to stop the spread of contagion. The alternative attitudes that Florentines adopted—utter abstemiousness and complete social isolation; carnal decadence and abandonment of law and order; irrational, panic-driven flight from village to village (52–53)—all have the same tragic end. These attitudes are the desperate gambits of those clinging to life itself as the highest good. The heroic resignation of the *Decameron* storytellers admits the likelihood that none will escape, admits the darkness of the hour, but nonetheless wills to take delight in small pleasures as long as life continues. The *Decameron* embraces humor because humor is an innocent pleasure that makes life better. This is the attitude of the tragicomic and the deathbed discourse of Socrates. This is stoicism, which is the most rational philosophy in dark times. Boccaccio's enduring message in times of pandemic is a playful and comical species of Stoic wisdom: *do not abandon the small pleasures of the everyday, and do not lose your sense of humor.*

Boccaccio's application of classical philosophical principles is part of his greatness as a humanist writer. In his own time and for many years after, his literary works were very little known outside of Italy. He was revered elsewhere not as a literary artist, but as a scholar of antiquity. Jacob

6 Epictetus, *The Discourses*, in *Discourses and Selected Writings*, trans. and ed. Robert Dobbin (New York: Penguin, 2008), I.i.22.

7 Lucius Annaeus Seneca, "On Providence," in *Dialogues and Essays*, trans. John Davie (New York: Oxford University Press, 2008), 4.

8 Ibid., "Consolation to Marcia," 57.

Burckhardt writes, "For two centuries, when but little was known of the 'Decameron' north of the Alps, he was famous all over Europe simply on account of his Latin compilations on mythology, geography and biography."[9] Guido Guarino says that "his *Genealogia Deorum Gentilium* in particular became the textbook and font of inspiration for generations of poets."[10] In keeping with the interests and projects of the humanists at the beginning of the Italian Renaissance, Boccaccio was deeply immersed in the newly rediscovered Greek and Latin classics. It was this renewed interest in the forgotten wisdom of the ancients that transformed the intellectual world of Europe in the fourteenth and fifteenth centuries and shattered the Roman Catholic Church's monopoly on thought. Boccaccio absorbed the lessons of the pagans and it opened his mind to viewpoints outside of the Roman Catholic paradigm, from which he was able to criticize and ridicule this paradigm and the many absurdities endemic to its officials (though without seriously questioning Christianity itself). The teachings of Socrates, Cicero, the Stoics, and others are lessons in *phronēsis*, or how to live well. These teachings are different from those of the Church. Often, the ancients employ a brilliant irony and humor that lightens the most somber moments. Socrates could be killed, but not made unhappy.

The middle ages were by no means humorless, but their humor was often of a wanton and irrational sort, reflecting the impotence of the common person to take action. The medieval Church held a hostile official position on laughter. St. Benedict condemned comic speech as sin in his *Rule for Monasteries*, and subjected laughter to a "perpetual ban."[11] The fanatic Jorge de Burgos in Umberto Eco's historical novel *The Name of the Rose* gives a long speech that reflects many medieval clerical views on laughter: "Laughter is weakness, corruption, the foolishness of our flesh. It is the peasant's entertainment, the drunkard's license," and so on.[12] An immersion in the ancient lightness of being gave Boccaccio the distance necessary to reject this Church doctrine. Boccaccio was the first great comic writer of the modern world, a master of satire both highbrow and

9 Jacob Burckhardt, *The Civilization of the Renaissance in Italy*, trans. S. G. C. Middlemore, rev. Ludwig Goldscheider (New York: Modern Library, 1995), 150.

10 Guido A. Guarino, Introduction to Boccaccio, *On Famous Women* (New York: Italica Press, 2011), ix.

11 See St. Benedict of Nursia, *St. Benedict's Rule for Monasteries*, trans. Leonard J. Doyle (Collegeville, MN: The Liturgical Press, 1950), ch. 4 (rules 54, 55), and ch. 6.

12 Umberto Eco, *The Name of the Rose*, trans. William Weaver (New York: Harcourt Brace & Company, 1984), 474–76.

lowbrow.[13] He was the intellectual ancestor of Rabelais, Swift, and Laurence Sterne. The importance of humor for the good life is a lesson that he learned not from his contemporaries, but from the vanquished pagan world of Juvenal and Petronius and Lucian.

There are two sorts of laughter. One is the vulgar laughter of those whose reason is impaired by either resentment, terror, or some other passion. The other is the delightful laughter of rational minds that know the true value of things and are sympathetic to the folly and delusion of unfortunate humans. Boccaccio presents these two forms of laughter as characteristic of two types of attitude toward the plague. He writes, "Few indeed were those to whom the lamentations and bitter tears of their relatives were accorded; on the contrary, more often than not bereavement was the signal for laughter and witticisms and general jollification—the art of which the women, having for the most part suppressed their feminine concern for the salvation of the souls of the dead, had learned to perfection" (55). This is the manic laughter and festival attitude of the hopeless, who have abandoned the good life. Those who laugh in this way do not demonstrate heroic victory over pain. They demonstrate only that fear has driven them to mistake the real value of things. They place their own immediate pleasure above basic humanity and sympathy. Significant losses *ought* to be mourned; it is only a fault when mourning exceeds its proper bounds. The wild laughter of the vulgar is the frenzied cult jubilation of the bacchants in Euripides, who delight in seeing a mother tear her son limb from limb. This sort of laughter does not add sweet pleasure to life; it debases life by undermining all value.

The second kind of laughter is that of Socrates. It is the innocent laughter of a soul that can see clearly the proper order of things. This is the laughter of persons who recognize their own folly and that of all others, and refuse to take themselves too seriously. It is the laughter of children, whose joy is simple and unmediated by desire. One of Boccaccio's young men says, "I know not what you intend to do with your troubles; my own I left inside the city gates when I departed thence a short while ago in your company. Hence you may either prepare to join with me in as much laughter, song and merriment as your sense of decorum will allow, or else you may give me leave to go back to my troubles and live in the afflicted city."

13 The contrast between Boccaccio and his contemporaries, particularly the romantic and serious Petrarch, is represented in literary form in Milan Kundera's novel, *The Book of Laughter and Forgetting*, trans. Aaron Asher (New York: HarperPerennial, 1999), 175–200.

One of the ladies responds, "There is much sense in what you say, Dioneo. A merry life should be our aim, since it was for no other reason that we were prompted to run away from the sorrows of the city" (64-65). It is rational deliberation on the good life that leads the characters to embrace levity and humor. They do not lie to themselves about the horrors of the surrounding world, but even recognizing these fully, they choose laughter over weeping and tearing out their hair as a more pleasant way to spend their time. This is not frivolity, but a profound spiritual victory over external fortune.

The stories that are told over the course of the fortnight of seclusion are not all comedic. Many are stories of love and loss, and some are stories with a moral lesson. However, the best known of these vignettes are infamous for their irreverence and bawdiness. Some satirize the excesses and abuses of monks and abbots, and the willing seduction of nuns (e.g. I.4, III.1, IX.2). Others involve the sexual games played between the men and women, wed and unwed (e.g. VIII.4, 7, 8). Charming tricksters place "a pair of horns upon His crown" (cuckold Christ by sleeping with his "brides") and suffer no misfortune (241). This irreverence is never irreligion, though. It is the hypocrisy and self-delusion of the proud that makes up the subject of Boccaccio's raillery. As Guido Guarino says, "Beneath all his laughter he remains a moralist."[14] The satires in the *Decameron* are meant to convey truths about human folly. We are all fools of different sorts, and true wisdom lies in recognizing our own folly. Satire of this sort teaches us self-knowledge. This is the lesson of Socrates' doctrine of ignorance and the *Characters* of Theophrastus. The theme of folly and self-delusion would run through later Renaissance literature, most notably Desiderius Erasmus' *In Praise of Folly* and Sebastian Brant's *Ship of Fools*. Brant describes the pedagogical benefit of portraying human folly:

> For fools a mirror shall it be,
> Where each his counterfeit may see.
> His proper value each would know,
> The glass of fools the truth may show.
> Who sees his image on the page
> May learn to deem himself no sage,
> Nor shrink his nothingness to see,
> Since none who lives from fault is free.[15]

14 Guarino, Introduction to *Famous Women*, xx.

15 Sebastian Brant, *The Ship of Fools*, trans. Edwin H. Zeydel (New York: Columbia University Press, 1944), 58.

Journey along the ship of fools and find the chamber where you belong.

I have argued elsewhere for the importance of humor as a philosophical instrument.[16] Humor shows the things of the world in ways that rational discourse does not. It juxtaposes serious persons with silly situations, or silly persons with serious situations. It throws things off balance and presents them in different lights, from different angles. It pulls down its target's pants; pulling down someone's pants reveals what is usually hidden and guarded. It empties out the pockets of grave men and tousles their hair, leaving them less fearsome. In doing so, it performs the work of the assayer. It tests raw ore and determines what in its constitution is gold and what is worthless. The sage uses humor as a divining rod.

The third Earl of Shaftesbury articulated the philosophical value of ridicule early in the eighteenth century. In his "*Sensus Communis*; an Essay on the Freedom of Wit and Humour," he writes, "Truth, 'tis supposed, may bear all lights; and one of those principal lights, or natural mediums, by which things are to be viewed, in order to a thorough recognition, is ridicule itself, or that manner of proof by which we discern whatever is liable to just raillery in any subject."[17] Raillery cannot be borne by hypocrites. The hypocrite stands on the false pretense of *gravitas* and demands that his or her work and character be taken entirely seriously. Hypocrites lack a doctrine of ignorance. Such people are fools who repress their own folly. For Shaftesbury, raillery is an invaluable instrument of discovery, a crucible of character. To ridicule something can do no harm if it holds up to this ridicule. More often, however, our emperors are revealed to have no clothes. The "important man" who bristles under criticism is undoubtedly a fraud. If I know myself to be in possession of a vibrant inner life, I can laugh at myself, whereas one who doubts this cannot. Seriousness is the last refuge of a scoundrel.

Shaftesbury's form of raillery is good-natured teasing subject to reason, rather than hilarity that holds reason in thrall. The latter would be buffoonery, which is the manic laughter of those enthralled by passion. As an instrument of reason, raillery has power both to enlighten and to please. Buffoonery, being inherently indiscriminating, only obfuscates truth and degrades one's sense of what is fine and what is base. The person who laughs at malicious insults has lost all understanding of value. Shaftesbury

16 See my *Shame, Fame, and the Technological Mentality* (Lanham, MD: Lexington, 2021), 145–52.

17 Anthony Ashley Cooper, third Earl of Shaftesbury, *Characteristics of Men, Manners, Opinions, Times*, ed. John M. Robertson (New York: Bobbs-Merrill, 1964), 44.

writes, "There is as much difference between one sort [of humor] and another as between fair-dealing and hypocrisy, or between genteel wit and the most scurrilous buffoonery."[18] Buffoonery keeps the mind immersed in its own pain and rage, whereas rational humor elevates the mind and lightens its troubles.

Boccaccio's lesson is that the rational species of humor and laughter are conducive to the good life, however tragic other conditions may be. Humor is pleasing and edifying, in the same way as a beautiful sunset or a kind gesture or good wine and song. Laughter is not itself the *summum bonum*, the final end of life, but it is always preferable and choice-worthy because it always adds to one's delight in life. As the Stoics teach, there is much over which individuals have no control. The plague that ravages one's entire world is one such thing. Laughter does not make one forget one's loss and pain. However, even under the dark cloud of loss of pain, laughter is still preferable to misery, just as even under the worst of conditions a rolling vista is still a sight preferable to a wasteland. Prudence, which is the art of living well, counsels us to embrace the simple pleasure of laughter when it comes, and to never take ourselves so seriously that we cannot see the absurdity of things.

The critical theorist Theodor Adorno once made a claim that has generated much discussion for nearly eighty years. He wrote, "Cultural criticism finds itself faced with the final stage of the dialectic of culture and barbarism. To write poetry after Auschwitz is barbaric."[19] Adorno's original meaning has been lost as this dictum has been repeated. Today, it is usually taken to mean that after the horrors of something as tragic and godless as the Holocaust, such enjoyments as poetry are frivolities. Boccaccio's contemporary, Petrarch, ran into this problem when he attempted to write about the Black Death: "Alas dearest brother, what shall I say? … Where are the magnificent words, which, if intended rather to extol your genius than as advice for life, can be no more than empty sounds and curious charms for the ears?"[20] The scale of the evil suffered by the human species is so enormous at times that little books of verse become meaningless and perhaps irresponsible. Is this so? If it is, then poetry is not alone. To eat a meal that is well seasoned must also be barbaric; to enjoy a child's soccer game must be barbaric. To laugh must be most barbaric of all, and

18 Ibid., 43.

19 Theodor W. Adorno, "Cultural Criticism and Society," in *Prisms*, trans. Samuel and Shierry Weber (Cambridge, MA: The MIT Press, 1983), 34.

20 Francesco Petrarch, *Letters on Familiar Matters*, trans. Aldo S. Bernardo (New York: Italica Press, 2005), VIII.7 [I:415].

must undermine the tragedy and suffering of human beings.

Humor, though, is neither barbaric nor frivolous. Seasoning one's meal does not keep one's body functioning any better, nor does it improve one's lot in life. Nevertheless, it should be practiced because well-seasoned dishes make one's meal a bit more pleasant. Eating unseasoned boiled chicken is not an evil and does no harm, but it does not tend to reaffirm life's delightfulness. Reading Yeats today does not undo the Holocaust, but it makes a world in which the Holocaust happened a little more pleasant for a moment. Laughter does not prevent the plague from striking and does not raise the rotting carcasses in the streets of Florence. However, it makes the moments between catastrophes a little more enjoyable. The prudence of the storytellers in the *Decameron* counsels them to choose jollity and laughter when it is available. Prudence today, in these dark and uncertain times, advises the same course. Laughter will not return the unemployed to work, nor will it cure the infected or raise those that have perished. However, we must never give up on living as well as we can, and that means feeling appropriate joy toward what is joyful. To give in to despair is to relinquish reason to the passions, which is acceptable only in moderation. Our happiest lives require us to seek a state of tranquility in which we can laugh when something is funny. To do so is to master all external evils and to live the lessons of the Stoics. To do so is to be Socrates, a joke on his lips with his final words.[21]

At the end of their fourteen days of isolation, the characters of the *Decameron* sacrifice their pleasant villa and decide the time is appropriate to return to Florence. This is presented as the demand of prudence: "The wisdom of mortals consists, as I think you know, not only in remembering the past and apprehending the present, but in being able, through a knowledge of each, to anticipate the future" (824). These are almost the very words used by Cicero in his description of the faculty of *prudentia*, prudence.[22] Boccaccio continues, "Accordingly, lest aught conducive to tedium should arise from a custom too long established, and lest, by protracting our stay, we should cause evil tongues to start wagging, I now think it proper … that with your consent we should return from whence we came" (825). The young ladies and gentlemen all agree to this course of action after deliberation. This shows that the laughter and gentle

21 For a longer account of the importance of humor for spiritual wellbeing, see my *Making Philosophy Laugh: Humor, Irony, and Folly in Philosophical Thought* (Eugene, OR: Cascade, 2023).

22 See Marcus Tullius Cicero, *De inventione*, trans. H. M. Hubbell (Cambridge, MA: Harvard University Press, 1949), II.liii.160.

pleasure of their retreat has not dulled their moral senses, nor deprived them of a sense of propriety and responsibility. Their laughter has remained subject to right reason, and when the moment is appropriate, reason counsels that the time for a return to Florence has come. Wit and humor do not undermine our self-control unless they descend into buffoonery. The young people resolve to return to the city of horrors, even knowing the high probability that doing so means rapid, painful death for themselves, because to stay away any longer would be imprudent. This is the final lesson of Boccaccio: humor is a fine and choice-worthy thing when appropriate, but it is only an adornment; it is not a substitute for substantive human action.

CHAPTER III

Lorenzo di Filippo Strozzi and Niccolò Machiavelli

An Epistle Written Concerning the Plague

Fall in Love to Escape the Deadly Plague

The Black Death of 1348 was the worst outbreak in the history of Florence, but it was by no means the city's only bubonic plague epidemic. Plague continued to flare up in Florence nearly once a decade until well into the seventeenth century. Particularly violent episodes struck in 1400, 1417, 1430, 1437, 1449, 1478, and 1527–31. Though none of these outbreaks had the enormous death toll of the Black Death, they were still formidable. The 1430 plague claimed around one fifth of Florence's population, and the outbreak of the late 1520s claimed one ninth. Apart from these major epidemics, there were also smaller outbreaks that occurred even more frequently, including one in the early 1520s.[1] The arts and sciences flourished in Florence during this time, as the small city became the epicenter of the Italian Renaissance. Good political minds like Coluccio Salutati and the enormous wealth of the Medici bankers drew Florence out of the middle ages and into modernity much earlier than much of Europe. Cultural giants like Pico della Mirandola, Girolamo Savonarola, da Vinci, Michelangelo, and Benvenuto Cellini called the city their home. Nevertheless, bubonic plague was a constant specter and an indomitable enemy.

The Florentine philosopher whose work has proven most enduring is Niccolò Machiavelli (1469–1527). Machiavelli's *The Prince* remains essential reading for political science students throughout the world. Machiavelli is much misunderstood and much maligned, and often taken as the prophet of amorality in politics. "Machiavellian" is a term for a cunning and unscrupulous person or action. This reputation already adhered to the man in his own century, as can be seen by the characterization of Machiavelli in Christopher Marlowe's *The Jew of Malta*:

> To some perhaps my name is odious,
> But such as love me guard me from their tongues;
> And let them know that I am Machiavel,

---

1 This data is from Alan S. Morrison, Julius Kirshner, and Anthony Molho, "Epidemics in Renaissance Florence," *American Journal of Public Health* 75 (1985): 528–35.

And weigh not men, and therefore not men's words.[2]

This view is not at all fair. *The Prince* openly advocates that, to remain in power, a prince must "learn to be able not to be good and to use this and not use it, according to necessity."[3] However, *The Prince* is a masterpiece of esoteric writing and irony, written with the deliberate intention of currying favor with the Medici family. Machiavelli had seen Girolamo Savonarola hanged and burned in the Piazza della Signoria, and had himself been exiled from Florence and tortured by *strappado* by the Medici family. He learned from these experiences the prudence of wearing different masks for different people. To view Machiavelli's character by an exoteric reading of *The Prince* is therefore to do little justice to the man.

Machiavelli was in fact an urbane and refined scholar and man of letters. Apart from his political tracts, he was an admirable historian and playwright, and his treatise on *The Art of War* was quite influential. He was engaged with Florentine politics in various roles throughout his life, and established the first Florentine militia. In his later life, he served as official historian of Florence. Like other Renaissance thinkers, Machiavelli's interests were quite diverse.

Despite living in a time of regular epidemics, Machiavelli seldom mentions bubonic plague in his writings. The exception is a curious manuscript in Machiavelli's hand entitled, *An Epistle Written Concerning the Plague* (*Pistola fatta per la peste*). Much about this letter remains unclear, but it was almost certainly not originally composed by Machiavelli himself. It was once thought to be an original composition, but its style is distinct from Machiavelli's other works, and the original of the manuscript has since been discovered. The primary author was one Lorenzo di Filippo Strozzi (1482–1547), a wealthy Renaissance polymath from a prominent Florentine banking family, who moved in the highest society of the day. Strozzi achieved success as a writer of histories, poems, and plays, and was considered a consummate gentleman. At the time of his death, Machiavelli possessed manuscripts of two of Strozzi's works, which he had copied out in his own hand: the *Epistle* and the *Commedia in versi*. The *Epistle* is peculiar in that the manuscript in Machiavelli's hand contains notations and corrections in Strozzi's hand. This has led to speculation that the work was either a collaboration between the two men, or that Machiavelli had

2 Christopher Marlowe, *The Jew of Malta*, ed. David Bevington (Manchester: Manchester University Press, 1997), lines 5–8.

3 Niccolò Machiavelli, *The Prince*, trans. Harvey C. Mansfield (Chicago: University of Chicago Press, 1998), 61.

an editorial role in its composition.[4]

The exact nature of the relationship between Strozzi and Machiavelli is unknown, though William Landon has convincingly argued that it was that of client and patron. A letter written in March of 1520 to Strozzi by his younger brother Filippo "expressed how pleased he was that Lorenzo had ushered Machiavelli into the good graces of Giulio de' Medici."[5] This suggests that Strozzi was instrumental in reconciling the disgraced Machiavelli with his enemies, the Medici, which Machiavelli was unable to accomplish himself through his dedication of *The Prince* to Lorenzo de' Medici. Machiavelli dedicated *The Art of War* to Strozzi in 1521 in fawning words that further suggest a client-patron relationship: "I inscribe it to you not only as a testimony of my gratitude, although conscious how small a return it is for favors I have received from you, but because it is usual to address things of this nature to persons who are distinguished by their nobility, riches, great talent, and generosity; I know very well that in birth and wealth you have not many equals, still fewer in talent, and in generosity, none at all."[6]

Landon writes, "Despite all this, as noted previously, one should not be tempted to conclude that Strozzi and Machiavelli were 'friends.' There is nothing anywhere in either man's work to indicate that their connection was anything other than professional."[7] For unknown reasons, Strozzi took an interest in Machiavelli and supported him as an advocate at court, and perhaps also financially or otherwise. However, the formality of Machiavelli's praise of the generous and talented Strozzi speaks more to indebtedness than friendship. Having been patronized by Strozzi, Machiavelli would have been obligated to fulfill certain tasks that Strozzi demanded. The transcription of the *Commedia* and the *Epistle* may have been a favor, or may have been a compulsory duty. Machiavelli may have served as an amanuensis for Strozzi, and seems to have contributed material for the composition of the *Epistle*. Certain passages resonate with the style and content of Machiavelli's other writings.

The *Epistle* is not, however, a literary or philosophical masterpiece,

---

4 On the history of the *Epistle*, as well as scholarly views on its composition and a brief life of Strozzi, see William J. Landon, *Lorenzo di Filippo Strozzi and Niccolò Machiavelli: Patron, Client, and the* Pistola fatta per la peste (Toronto: University of Toronto Press, 2013).

5 Ibid., 8.

6 Machiavelli, *The Art of War*, trans. Ellis Farneworth, rev. Neal Wood (Cambridge, MA: Da Capo, 2001), 5.

7 Landon, *Strozzi and Machiavelli*, 20.

and does not measure up to Machiavelli's other writings. In whatever degree of collaboration it was composed, its primary author was certainly Strozzi. The theme of the *Epistle* is romantic love. This is not a theme often associated with Machiavelli, and romance plays little role in his political writings. However, it is a topic that was often on his mind. The plots of his comedies *Mandragola* and *Clizio* revolve around erotic love and its foibles (as does the *Andria*, which Machiavelli translated from Terence). In his correspondence, Machiavelli reveals a susceptibility to erotic desire:

> So [Cupid], full of indignation and fury,
> in order to give proof of his exalted excellence,
> changed quiver, changed arrow and bow;
> and he fired one with such violence
> that I still grieve over my wounds,
> and I confess and acknowledge his power.[8]

The erotic romance of the *Epistle* is more in keeping with Strozzi's usual rakish style, but Machiavelli likely had something to contribute.

Whatever the truth behind the authorship of the *Epistle*, the more pertinent matter is whether it can teach us anything today. The lesson that we may extract from this short letter is that *love makes pandemics more bearable, and romance can still be kindled even during an outbreak.*

The *Epistle* purports to be an authentic letter from one friend to another, giving a "true" narration of a day in plague-ravaged Florence. Its addressee is Girolamo di Maestro Luca, who we are told has sensibly retreated from Florence to his villa in the country. The author feels compelled to give a report on plague conditions to his friend. Concerning his motive for writing, he says, "While [this letter] proves to you that I (of whose death perhaps you have heard) might yet live, it also will oblige you to make less grave every melancholy or other painful nuisance" (177).[9] This suggests from the beginning that the narrative of the letter will be comic, and will serve like the tales of the *Decameron* to distract and lighten the mind.

None of this is genuine, however. The letter was seemingly composed in 1522, during one of the rare periods when Florence was not enveloped by plague. Between 1479 and 1527, Florence was free from

---

8 Letter to Francesco Vettori (Aug. 1514), qtd. and trans. in John M. Najemy, *Between Friends: Discourses of Power and Desire in the Machiavelli—Vettori Letters of 1513–1515* (Princeton, NJ: Princeton University Press, 1993), 326.

9 All parenthetical citations in this section refer to Landon's translation of *An Epistle Concerning the Plague Year*, in *Strozzi and Machiavelli*, 174–209 (Italian and English on facing pages).

serious epidemics. There were occasional minor outbreaks, but nothing on the scale of the scenes of devastation presented in the *Epistle*'s narrative.[10] During the last serious outbreak, which claimed 4,000 souls in 1478, Machiavelli had been a child, and Strozzi was not yet born. That this plague narrative is an authentic report on conditions is thus an obvious playful deception. This also undermines the idea that it was genuinely intended as an informative letter to a friend. During the Renaissance, the two most characteristic literary forms were the oration and the epistle. The epistle received new literary life in Europe after the letters of Cicero were rediscovered and their form was widely imitated. The *Epistolae familiares* of Petrarch belong to this class of composition. It was common practice to use the epistolary form for expressing ideas for mass consumption.

The description of the plague given in the *Epistle* is not drawn from the personal experience of its authors, but is largely borrowed from both the collective memory of the Florentines and the introduction to Boccaccio's *Decameron.* Machiavelli strongly approved of Boccaccio's description in his *Florentine Histories*, speaking there of "that memorable pestilence celebrated with such eloquence by Messer Giovanni Boccaccio."[11] In the *Epistle*, Strozzi (or Machiavelli) writes, "One finds that our miserable Florence, at the present, resembles a city that has been sacked by the infidels and afterwards abandoned. Some of the inhabitants, such as yourself, have retired to country villas to escape the deadly plague; some are dead and others are approaching death; so that the whole present circumstances offend us, the future threatens us, so as one struggles with death, one fears for one's life." The streets of the city "are now stinking, ugly and swarming with the poor. One passes by their impudent and fearful shrieks with trepidation. The shops are locked, the businesses closed, the courts and the lawyers dragged away, prostrating the laws. Now one hears of this theft, not of that murder." As this nihilistic crime erupts, even the most intimate bonds are compromised: "Even if one parent finds the other, or a brother finds his brother, or a wife her husband, each one keeps a safe distance from their relations: and what is worse? Fathers and mothers spurn their children, abandoning them" (179–81).

The universal suffering of the city is vividly depicted. This description of the general condition of Florence betokens a grim tale to follow. However, the narration that actually follows is by turns surreal, comical, and erotic. It defies any attempt at pigeonholing into a literary genre. It has

10 Morrison et al., "Epidemics," 530.
11 Machiavelli, *Florentine Histories*, 104.

aspects of the picaresque, but could be called a *Bildungsroman* in brief, a novel of character development that takes place over the course of a single day (similar to Herman Melville's *Confidence Man*). We see the narrator's values and his views on romance change dramatically in the course of his wanders through the ghastly city.

Strozzi offers this day in his life as the measure of how all Florentines live during the plague. He writes, "The thing imagined compared with the truth of that which one imagines never adds up. Nor am I able, it seems to me, to illustrate this with a finer example than my own life: therefore I will describe my life to you, so that by it you may measure all the rest" (183). This claim mirrors Michel de Montaigne's justification for taking himself as the subject of his *Essays*: "I offer a humble and inglorious life; that does not matter. You can tie up all moral philosophy with a common and private life just as well as with a life of richer stuff. Each man bears the entire form the human condition [*l'humaine condition*]."[12] Because Strozzi is simply a human being subject to the same conditions as others, his experience is a microcosm of general experience. However, the uniqueness of his narration proves this to be a tongue-in-cheek claim. Over the course of a single day, the narrator visits nearly all of the major churches of Florence, has multiple sexual encounters, and ends up betrothed to a beautiful young widow. Presumably, a sudden engagement to a stranger is not typical of the human condition even in times of plague.

In the early morning of a work day, Strozzi leaves his home "before that hour in which all the terrestrial vapors are evaporated by the sun." Naturally, he first encounters gravediggers. The gravediggers are aggrieved neither by the horrors of the pestilence nor the risk to themselves of infection, but by the prospect of a future scarcity of bodies, "that such an abundance begets their future famine" (183). The first church at which he stops is the Duomo, where there are only six elderly parishioners, three old men who are lasciviously "giving the eye" to three "old bent and perhaps lame women." One of the three priests in the Duomo is shackled at wrists and ankles, to "better escape temptations in canonical solitude" (185–87). These scenes and others of the same sort are permeated by black humor, and the wandering narrator who passes from church to church interprets his surroundings with a lusty eye and a cynic's wit.

At Santa Croce (the basilica that today houses the tomb of Machiavelli), after passing by merrymaking gravediggers who dance and sing "Hearty welcome, plague," the narrator comes upon a prostrate young

12 Montaigne, *Complete Essays*, 631.

lady, distraught and rending her own hair. The plague has recently taken her "ill-fated, faithful lover," to whom she was bound by "the indissoluble lovers' knot, which so much of my artistry and diligence fabricated." The "fabrication" of this knot suggests learned mastery in the arts of seduction, and we will see that this young man was not her only ensnared lover. She is something like a "companion," or what the Greeks called a *hetaera*. She mourns not for the loss of her lover's spiritual qualities, but rather laments with great sensuality, "Oh what pleasure when I pressed my longing lips to his fragrant mouth! Oh with such great contentment I united and squeezed my burning breasts to his warm and pure and youthful chest! Oh wretched me! So frequently and with such bliss we came to that final amorous joy, simultaneously slaking our desires!" (191). The narrator's lustiness emerges, and we encounter his tendency toward sexual aggression and indecency. To "comfort" the mourner, he writes, "I, with that carnal affection that requires it, lightly began to caress her body; unlacing her dress in front, although she was not very tightly laced," and so on, all of this at the altar of Santa Croce. He proceeds to convince her "not for love of me, for I am unworthy of it, to come with me; for the sake of your honor, which, will be entirely restored. ... Because, I know many women who fled from their husbands, sheltering with others than their parents" (193–95). He gently urges, "Sin certainly is a human thing" (195), escorting her to her home, where the pair presumably share the bed of the late deceased.

Strozzi's attitude toward sex at this point in the tale is cavalier and immoral. He readily takes what advantage he can seize, and cares nothing for romance or spiritual eroticism. These characteristics are emphasized just as much in the next encounter he has, at the church of Santa Trinità. Here, he meets a well-born man of means, and he asks the man why he has remained in Florence rather than fleeing like so many others. The man's initial pretense is that he has remained for love of his native city. When the narrator presses the issue, the man finally admits, "If I must tell the truth to one who knows it already, it is not our native city that keeps me here, but it is that disconsolate lady who you saw so devotedly genuflecting—for whose love I am prepared to lay down my life" (197). It is unclear how the man would know of Strozzi's earlier encounter, but this is evidence that he is yet another gentleman who has been seduced by the young lady. Clearly, his affections for her are not reciprocal, as she beds Strozzi and pines for the embraces of a third man.

"Such is the degree of my love, that it surpasses every type of blood relation," the man continues. "If to avoid the plague to be happy is an excellent remedy, then to be in the presence of her love was tremendous joy, and away from her love such grief that it alone would cause him to depart this life bitterly and alone as he was found here … and he concluded by saying that being in love, and wishing to live, that I should remain close to my lover. Not being so yet, but moved by his example, he urged me to fall in love to escape the deadly plague; and told me that I still had time" (197).

This is a confession of passionate, emotional *eros*. Such *eros* involves more of the entire self than the carnal, sensual *eros* that aims only at bodily gratification. The man is a fool, because he fails to recognize the inequality in his love for the lady, and invests the relationship with much more significance than it has for her. He sees her love as his *salvation*, whereas her motives are mercenary and utilitarian. It is a skilled courtesan that binds both body and mind. He has invested the wrong person with his lofty sentiments, which is folly and delusion. However, those sentiments themselves are not folly. There is a lesson to be learned from this man, though Strozzi is not yet equipped to internalize his counsel. *Eros* is divine, as the ancients knew well, and to sacrifice one's human interest for divine goods is laudable. The man remains in Florence because he yearns, and that is something. For what reason does Strozzi remain, hazarding death? Why stroll without aim or purpose from one end of the city to the other? In what things does the young wastrel find meaning? Without asking himself these questions, he jests, "I was not persuaded by these arguments, judging love a much more dangerous and longer lasting pestilence" (197).

The humanist idea of love that flourished in Renaissance thought was largely derived from the Platonic notion of *eros*. In Plato's *Symposium*, Socrates describes love as a spiritual project, in the image of a ladder. The lover "goes always upwards for the sake of this Beauty, starting out from beautiful things and using them like rising stairs."[13] The initiate in erotics first falls in love with the beauty of a particular body. Reflection shows that the particular features he finds beautiful are common to many bodies, and he learns to see beauty in all bodies. He next realizes that what gives bodies their beauty is that they suggest beauty of soul, which is another rung ascended. At the apex of the ladder, the love of particular individuals has transformed into a love of love itself. Progress in erotics carries one from the particular to the general, from the concrete to the abstract, from the physical to the spiritual. Love of individual beauties is only the first step toward love of the form of Beauty itself. This idea of *eros* as

13 Plato, *Symp.*, 211c.

spiritual development was Italianized and popularized in Renaissance Florence through the teaching of Marsilio Ficino, founder of the Florentine Academy. Ficino attempted to synthesize Christianity and Platonism in his *Platonic Theology*. Here, Plato's ladder of love becomes a pious work. Ficino writes that the degree of clarity of the divine substance "comes to our minds from the diverse degrees of love, and with those degrees—and not unjustly so—diverse degrees of vision and still more so of joy coincide."[14] Brian Copenhaver writes that Ficino successfully persuaded the Florentine public that "love between embodied individuals is a secondary but valued effect of the love of each person for God, toward whom all souls finally converge."[15]

This idea of a higher, spiritual love was by no means universal in Florence or elsewhere, but it was the dominant form in which *eros* was portrayed in the literature of the day. Dante's pure love for Beatrice carries him to Paradiso, where even Virgil may not follow. The chaste, spiritual love of Petrarch shines throughout his *Canzoniere*. There were always writers like Pietro Aretino whose notion of love was much more carnal, but such literati were outnumbered within the highest intellectual circles of Florence. Machiavelli, an excellent classicist, was deeply attuned to the Platonic notion of *eros* (though his personal letters occasionally show a scatological humor), and Strozzi was no doubt familiar with Ficino's doctrine of Platonic love.

The Platonic ideal of love plays an unusual role in the *Epistle*. The reason I characterize the letter as a *Bildungsroman* is because the narrator seems to develop in the field of erotics. However imperfect his ascent of the latter of love, the movement is still upward, and beginning from pure sensualism, he arrives at higher rung. Amid descriptions of the gravediggers' festival and occasional corpses along the bridges, the *Epistle* contains three scenes that deal with love. The first, we have seen, is completely carnal. Strozzi and the young lady in mourning are attracted bodily to one another. They copulate and then part without another thought for one another. The "art" of their coupling is an art of physical gratification. The beauty of the lady's body does not inspire spiritual development. The second scene is the conversation with this lady's other lover, who lauds *eros* in the Platonic or Ficinian manner, however naïve he may be. His folly

14 Marsilio Ficino, *Platonic Theology*, trans. Michael J. B. Allen (Cambridge, MA: Harvard University Press, 2006), XVIII.viii.27.

15 Brian P. Copenhaver and Charles B. Schmitt, *Renaissance Philosophy* (New York: Oxford University Press, 1992), 144.

shows that he is not a true philosopher, and that his understanding of erotics is imperfect. Though he has fine ideals, he has not applied them correctly. There is nonetheless a kernel of truth in what he says. Strozzi mocks his advice, but will come close to the man's attitude in short order. The first encounter takes place in the morning, the second at midday, and the final encounter is in the evening. The passing of the day represents the development of Strozzi's spiritual maturity.

The third scene is the climax of the narration. The final church the narrator visits is the Santa Maria Novella. He is attracted to this basilica because he is told that "more ladies than one could wish for were assembled there (perhaps owing to the amorous instruction of the festive and charitable brothers)." This is told to him by a venerable friar, excluded from Santa Maria "for his good behavior" (199). This church is painted as a bacchic sanctuary for the lusty, a place where men of God initiate young women into the cult of Venus, a church that excludes religion. Naturally, Strozzi hastens to services there. By this time, it is the Compline hour (around seven in the evening), the end of the ecclesiastical day.

At Santa Maria, Strozzi beholds a beautiful young woman in widow's clothing. He describes her as being "of an agreeable size and proportionate stature for a finely formed woman. So that even from here one could conclude that all the parts of such a body were so well shaped, that if stripped of her mourning raiment, they would present a wondrous beauty to my eyes. … Her smooth and tender skin resembles spotless ivory yet so soft and delicate as to preserve the traces of even the lightest touch." In her eyes, "one saw paradise opened" (201). More of this kind follows, her breasts being two apples grown in the garden of the Hesperides, and her hands of such virtue that they would arouse aged Priam (205). Landon refers to such flourishes as "learned pornography,"[16] though they are tame and sophisticated by modern standards.

Interspersed with these "pornographic" reflections, Strozzi evinces a double attraction. He notes that her physiognomy suggests "acute prudence [*prudenzia*] or intelligence" (203). Prudence, we have seen, is knowledge of right action and living well. This is not a virtue often found desirable by the seducer. Further, the lady's visage in the work of two goddesses: "From Juno, she has a delicately formed nose, as from Venus that of her playful and flowery cheeks" (203). Venus is the erotic deity, but Juno is the goddess who sanctifies commitment and watches over the marital hearth. Giambattista Vico writes, "The theological poets who had

16 Landon, *Strozzi and Machiavelli*, 11.

created the divine character of Jove now created a second, that of solemn matrimony; namely, Juno, the second divinity of the so-called greater gentes." Juno derives from "*jugalis*, 'of the yoke,' with reference to the yoke of solemn matrimony."[17] Solemn matrimony is one of the basic principles of human civilization. It is Venus that attracts Strozzi, but after this initial attraction, more noble thoughts emerge. The lady speaks in terms resonant of Juno, not Venus, when approached by the narrator (unlike his earlier conquest). "Why do you stay here so alone?" asks Strozzi, suggesting that she take solace in an extramarital liaison. She responds, "Because I alone am spared, must I have a husband in order to please you? I wish for nothing more than to live married honestly" (207). She is a devotee of divinely solemnized marriage, which is a civic rite, rather the wanton profligacy of barbarians.

This brings about the narrator's sudden change of position on *eros*. Previously, he jested that love was more frightful and harmful than the plague itself. He now revisits this assertion: "I, who before this moment never wished to marry a woman, now see your beautiful and gracious form, upon whom Nature bestowed its bounty, and moved to compassion by your afflictions, am resolved to marry you." When she accuses him of being insincere, he pleads, "One who knows how to choose prudently does not have to put his faith in the truthfulness of others and therefore never has to repent of what he has done" (207). The two leave together for her home, where "together with my heart, she locked herself. From whence I departed alone, so happy and intensely delighted by my sweet wife." After sharing nuptial intimacy, Strozzi is overpowered by a new emotion and, "as those who taste of the river Lethe, I forgot every other woman, however lovely" (209). Lethe is the river of oblivion, in which the whole of the past is forgotten and one enters life anew. The experience described here is a Dantesque *vita nuova*, the inauguration of a new life with a new ordering of values. Strozzi's final words show this shift of paradigm: "putting an ending to this tragic consideration of the horrendous plague, I prepare myself for the pleasure of a future comedy for the following evening" (209).

The shift from tragedy to comedy comes about through the mediation of this new, solemn form of *eros*. It is an old commonplace that tragedies end with a funeral, while comedies end with a wedding. The narrator's existence is transformed from a solitary, aimless life of wandering, copulating, and story-telling, which sociability can end only in his funeral, to a faithful life sanctified by heaven, in which spiritual beauty is admired as much bodily beauty. His forthcoming wedding takes the place of his likely

17 Vico, *New Science*, §§512, 513.

death. The date of this narration is purportedly the first of May, the traditional spring holiday. May Day is the festival of generation, celebrating the return of growth and fertility out of the long months of barrenness. Strozzi undergoes the same sort of ritual transformation, corresponding with his ascent from the bottom rung of the ladder of love to a higher position. He is not yet Socrates; he is still deeply immersed in sensual delights. However, the oblivion of the past has begun, and from beauties of the flesh, he has taken a step upward for the sake of that beauty. Ultimately, the narrator arrives at a version of Ficino's model of love, diluted with worldly realism and free from the idealism of Ficino and the naiveté of the foolish man in Santa Trinità.

The lesson for us to internalize from this epistle is that taught by the fool the narrator meets: "Fall in love to escape the deadly plague," for you still have time. Pandemics are tragedies, which bring universal suffering and distress, and end in funerals. However, until we are the ones interred, it always remains possible to make comedy out of tragedy. "Hearty welcome, plague" becomes "Hearty welcome, May." We may evolve, we may discover new purpose and alight upon new values or arrange our values in new orders. An erotic attraction that elevates one to a loftier position on the ladder of love brings forgetfulness for the troubles of the body. Through Platonic love, the mind's focus is shifted from concern with the physical to the ideal. When thought is elevated to a more spiritual plane, the pestilence that ravages corporeal flesh weighs less heavily. *Eros* transforms suffering into festival, winter into spring. Love of this type is sanctioned under the auspices of Juno.

If we absorb the *Epistle* of Signori Strozzi and Machiavelli (however ironic, rakish, and even pornographic this letter may be), we discover that it counsels us to cultivate erotic life even during times of pestilence. Spiritual meditations are therapy for bodily worries, and the comedy of marriage is the best inoculation against the tragedy of pandemics. Today, there are countless ways to discover romance even amongst the quarantined. The mediation of technology has made physical proximity much less significant than it was in the Florence of the Medici. Sitting alone lamenting our misfortune is not encouraged by any classical notion of the good life. Prudence demands that we continue to look for love even in the time of cholera.

CHAPTER IV

François Rabelais

Gargantua and Pantagruel

Plague is Not Divine Punishment

François Rabelais (1494–1553) was a physician and medical teacher by trade, prior to becoming one of the most well-known and influential humanist writers of the French Renaissance. Already a Franciscan priest and monk, he completed his medical studies in Paris and Montpellier during the 1520s and early '30s, and spent two years as a doctor in the large Hôtel-Dieu hospital in Paris. In 1534, he was called to Rome to serve as physician to the Bishop of Paris, Jean du Bellay. While there, he impressed the pope with his medical skill. He took advanced medical degrees at Montpellier later in the decade and lectured there on Hippocrates. He later spent two years as physician and secretary to Guillaume, seigneur de Langey, the governor of Turin and du Bellay's older brother.[1]

At this time, the ancient doctrines and assumptions of Greek medicine were being overthrown in favor of more empirical forms of investigation. Physicians no longer accepted on authority the principles of Galen and Hippocrates that had been foundational to western medicine for centuries. Their four "qualities" of hot, cold, moist, and dry, "to the operation of [which] is due the genesis and destruction of all things that come into and pass out of being,"[2] failed to survive the rigors of the new sciences emerging in Renaissance Europe. Trish Nicholson writes, "Under humanist influence, medical schools were beginning to question the thousand-year-old wisdom of Galen and Hippocrates on which their teaching was based. Legally and illegally, corpses were being dissected, and enlightened individuals began giving direct observation more credence over ancient theory." Leonardo da Vinci was a notable proponent of these methods. Ibn al-Nafis had already deciphered the circulation of blood in animals, and

1 See the short biography of Rabelais by Donald M. Frame in the Introduction to Frame's translation of *The Complete Works of François Rabelais* (Los Angeles: University of California Press, 1999), esp. xxix–xxxi. All parenthetic references in this section refer to this text.

2 Aelius Galen, *On the Natural Faculties*, trans. Arthur John Brock (Cambridge, MA: Harvard University Press, 2006), I.ii.

Arabic discoveries in medicine were beginning to influence European physicians. Rabelais embraced the new observational approach to medicine; he was "keenly interested in these new developments and no doubt applied them when he could. In recognition, the Pope appointed Rabelais a secular priest, allowing him to travel more freely."[3]

This medical training and practice gave Rabelais a more intimate and technical knowledge of pathology and epidemiology than most other literary figures who have written on the topic. Rabelais' first encounter with plague came during his travels, when he was prevented by an outbreak from entering Tours. He had occasion to treat plague victims, at the risk of his own life, during his time as a physician in Paris and Rome, as Europe was still in the midst of the devastating "Second Plague Pandemic." However, because the Black Death with which this pandemic began had so ravaged the continent, "fear of the plague and an array of social reactions to it had become just as common and harmful, though not as deadly, as the sickness itself."[4] Fear is the mother of superstition, which is the attempt to make sense of phenomena whose power and source we do not comprehend. Superstition is a reversion to mythical thinking, which we discussed in dealing with Thucydides.

Rabelais composed his comic masterpiece, *Gargantua and Pantagruel*, in five volumes over the course of the last two decades of his life (roughly 1532–53). The writing of the book coincides with much of his time as a practicing physician. As a matter of course, the omnipresent specter of the plague and the popular fears about infection, both rational and irrational, felt by many Europeans, made their way into his narrative.

When Rabelais acknowledges plague, it is usually with the satirical and burlesque wit of an intellectual descendent of Boccaccio. He narrates a description of the inside of the giant Pantagruel's mouth as though describing a geographic region of the world. Here, in the cities of Larynx and Pharynx ("two large cities such as Rouen and Nantes, rich and doing good business"), plague has devastated the populations. "People near here are dying so fast that the tumbrel keeps running through the streets." What has caused this terrible inter-oral outbreak? "The cause of the plague was a foul stinking exhalation that had issued from the gulfs not long ago, from which over twenty-two hundred and sixty thousand and sixty persons have

---

3 Trish Nicholson, *A Biography of Story, a Brief History of Humanity* (Leicestershire: Matador, 2016), 259–60.

4 Elizabeth Chesney Zegura, ed., *The Rabelais Encyclopedia* (Westport, CT: Greenwood, 2004), art. "Plague," 189.

died in a week. Then I thought and calculated, and decided it was a stinking breath that had come from Pantagruel's stomach when he ate all that garlic sauce" (240).

In another narration, Rabelais characterizes the dispositions of Pantagruel's erudite and cunning companion, Panurge (literally, "knave"). Panurge is said to have had the utmost contempt for Parisian scholars. On one occasion, "he made a mud-pie composed of lots of garlics, galbanum, asafoetilda, and castoreum, of good warm turds, and steeped it in ooze from pocky sores; and very early in the morning he greased and anointed the whole pavement with it, so that the devil himself could not have stood it." This procedure led to an outbreak of myriad diseases amongst the scholars. "All these fine folk were throwing their guts up in front of everybody, as if they had flayed the fox: and ten or twelve of them died of the plague, fourteen were lepers, eighteen were goutie, and over twenty-seven got the pox from it. But he didn't worry the least bit about it" (187).

In both of these scenes, Rabelais acknowledges the terrible deadliness of plague, while at the same time transforming this deadliness into an article of raillery. People who are infected with plague die, and in fact large numbers of people die in this way. Over two million lives are lost in Pantagruel's mouth in one week alone. Rabelais the worldly physician does not show any desire to whitewash the medical reality of plague conditions. However, he is also turning the grim threat of the plague on its head. This terribly fatal pandemic occurs inside of a mouth, and is caused by the belching of garlic sauce. The outbreak amongst the Parisian scholars is deliberately caused by the scatological pranks of a rogue. To turn something on its head is to show it in a comical light. The serious person suddenly appears a fool when he or she is turned upside down and shaken, pockets emptying and hair flying wildly asunder. Likewise, the serious pandemic is made laughable when turned upside down. Satire does not make the plague any less deadly, but it makes it less frightful. This too, the satirist shows, is absurd; this too is silly. We are reminded: "Vanity of vanities! All is vanity."[5] The pitched tension of fear that blights the healthy is taught to find what is laughable in its hobgoblin. By teaching us to laugh, Rabelais turns a mirror upon our own folly and our own seriousness, and offers us catharsis.

In these two vignettes, plague is treated incidentally, as a narrative device, but elsewhere in the book Rabelais offers direct reflections upon plague. As has already been said, the actual medical harm done by the

5 Ecc. 1:2.

pandemic was compounded by the superstitious fears of common, uneducated Europeans. This dread, liable to rise to the level of religious panic, causes a great deal of harm. Large-scale outbreaks always lead to some level of mass panic and hysteria while medical technicians have not yet developed efficient treatments.[6] Another man of letters, Jack London, portrays a scene one can well imagine: "The panic outrush for the country began. Imagine, my grandsons, people, thicker than the salmon-run you have seen on the Sacramento river, pouring out of the cities by millions, madly over the country, in vain attempt to escape the ubiquitous death."[7] Panic is the blind terror caused by Pan, who frightens mortals out of their wits with nighttime woodland noises. It is irrational and unreflective, and persons under the guidance of panic are unable to judge soundly. When reason does not have mastery of the self, the normal mechanisms of self-preservation and care for one's community malfunction. Panic both impedes those actions that are necessary for safety and inspires other actions that put one in the way of danger. During pandemics, *self-control* is the one thing needful.

There is a long tradition of humans ascribing plagues and pestilences to divine punishment. We have seen that the ancient pagans popularly held this belief, although Thucydides did not. Just as frequently, monotheistic Scripture associates the outbreak of plague with divine punishment for mortal iniquities. "Let my people go, so that they may worship me. For this time I will send all my plagues upon you yourself, and upon your officials, and upon your people." "The anger of the Lord was kindled against the people, and the Lord struck the people with a very great plague." "And I will send sword, famine, and plague upon them, until they are utterly destroyed from the land that I gave them and their ancestors." "I will cut you down; my eye will not spare, and I will have no pity. One third of you shall die of plague or be consumed by famine among you." "We sent on the transgressors a plague from heaven, for that they infringed (our command) repeatedly."[8] In all of these passages, the sins of mortals are chastised by the divine through plague. If pandemics are caused by the wrath of God, mortal sinners have no hope of mitigation through human ingenuity. In such situations, the only means of averting disaster is repentance,

6 See Mark Honigsbaum, *The Pandemic Century: One Hundred Years of Panic, Hysteria, and Hubris* (New York: W. W. Norton, 2019) on the persistence of this phenomenon in the twentieth century.

7 Jack London, *The Scarlet Plague* (New York: Macmillan, 1915), 89.

8 Exod. 9:13-14; Num. 11:33; Jer. 24:10; Ezek. 5:12; Qu'ran 2:59. The last refers to *The Holy Qur'an*, trans. Abdullah Yusuf Ali (Hertfordshire: Wordsworth, 2000).

which is the particular theme of the prophetic books of Scripture.

Rabelais, an enlightened man from an age of science, found such thinking counter-productive. If no better solution presents itself, it is acceptable to embrace the paradigm imagined by religious dread. However, if there are steps that human beings can take to prevent and fight against disease, then humanism demands that these steps be taken. The religious view of the plague is an obstacle to the practical steps necessary for medical intervention, which require the cooperation of the masses and coordinated action. The lesson taught by Rabelais, when he speaks categorically about the plague rather than using it as a comic device, is that *the plague is not divine punishment, and superstitious behavior expedites the damage.* It is a natural phenomenon, with natural, worldly causes. Pandemics are nothing supernatural.

Gargantua, the first novel of the *Gargantua and Pantagruel* collection, was published in 1532, and written while Rabelais was a serving as a doctor at the Hôtel-Dieu. *Gargantua* contains two chapters that argue against the idea of plague being divine punishment. In Chapter 27, the city of Seville is attacked and plundered by enemies during an outbreak of plague. Rabelais writes, "Although the plague was there throughout most of the houses, they went in everywhere, plundered all that was inside, and never did one of them run any danger, which is a pretty marvelous thing; for the curates, vicars, preachers, physicians, surgeons, and apothecaries who went to examine, bind up, cure, preach to, and admonish the sick had all died of the infection, and those pillaging and murderous devils never got ill. How does that come about? Think about it, I beg you" (65). Plague is indiscriminate and does not distinguish the pious from the impious, or the good from the evil. Rabelais shows us that God does not use disease as a chastisement of the wicked. Taken as a natural contagion, the plague does not require the composition of a subtle theodicy. No Leibniz is necessary, nor a Voltaire to laugh at him. However, if we believe that plague is God's punishment, and we must explain why it disproportionately kills decent human beings, the practical lesson becomes lost beneath sophistical quibbling.

What is the practical lesson that Rabelais suggests with his "Think about it"? Under siege conditions, people retreat as much as possible from pillagers and burglars. When an armed and belligerent enemy is within our home, we hide if at all possible; if not, we barricade ourselves in the most secure location. Physical confrontation is avoided, especially if disease has impeded our bodily faculties. Retreat is the rule in such situations. Further, the objects stolen by thieves are not objects that infected persons regularly handle—jewelry, candlesticks, artworks, and so on. Not so with angels of mercy. The physician who tends to our sores; the clergyman who sits and prays with us; the nurse who lays cool hands on our feverish heads—this proximity is the cause of transmission of the illness. It is physical contact that passes contagion from one body to another, not targeted divine wrath. The benevolent friend that we embrace is much more likely to fall victim to our contagion than the hostile enemy from whom we recede. At the center of the psychology of children is the principle that benign objects attract and malignant objects repulse. This is the most tragic aspect of pandemics, as we will see again with Daniel Defoe: loved ones become the scourge of one another.

Rabelais continues this analysis more substantially in Chapter 45. Here, Gargantua and his father Grandgousier encounter a group of pilgrims on their way to the shrine of Saint-Sébastien, near Nantes. When asked about the motive of their pilgrimage, one of their number says, "We are going to offer our prayers against the plague" (103). Grandgousier asks, "O, you poor folk, do you think the plague comes from Saint-Sébastien?" and the pilgrim responds, "Yes indeed, and our preachers assert it" (104). This addresses the complicity of religious authorities in the spurious religious superstitions of the masses. Popular superstition amongst uneducated peasants is sanctioned and enflamed by preachers who, Rabelais believes, act irresponsibly and ought to know better.

Grandgousier voices the outrage of Rabelais: "Do the false prophets [*faulx prophetes*] announce such abuses to you? Do they in this way so blaspheme God's just men and saints that they make them out like those devils who do nothing but harm among humans, as Homer writes that the plague was sent into the Greek host by Apollo, and as the poets invent a pile of Vedioves and other maleficent divinities? Thus one hypocrite at Sinay was preaching that Saint Anthony set fire to legs, Saint Eutropius made people dropsical, Saint Gildas made people mad, Saint Genou brought on the gout." Grandgoisier, as king, "made such an example of his punishment, although he called me a heretic, that from that time on not one hypocrite has dared to enter my lands." Thus, Rabelais suggests, should all false Jeremiahs and hypocritical preachers of divine punishment be punished by good monarchs. Grandgousier continues, "I am amazed if your king lets them preach such scandal in his kingdom; for they are more to be punished than those who by magical art or other device would have spread the plague around the country. The plague kills only the body, but such imposters poison souls" (104). At this point, the polemic is interrupted and the pilgrims do not respond.

There is much in the discourse of Grandgousier that is pertinent and edifying for us today. Most religious leaders have denied that the present outbreak is divine retaliation for human iniquity, but some have taken the opposite position. Both clerical and secular preachers (ranging from the pastors of some megachurches to wrestling legend Hulk Hogan) can easily be found who claim that COVID-19 is a chastisement aimed at this or that group for some particular set of sins. Pennsylvania state representative Stephanie Borowicz, for instance, recently called COVID-19 "a punishment inflicted upon us for our presumptuous sins" and attempted to pass a resolution declaring March 30 "a state day of humiliation, fasting and prayer in Pennsylvania."[9] What was true in the time of Thucydides remains true today: when people do not know or understand what has caused their ill fortune, they are inclined to look to the heavens and attribute it to higher powers. Meaningless and arbitrary suffering becomes more palatable (and even noble) if we impose sacred meaning upon it, and imagine a path within our grasp—namely, repentance—that can ensure our safety.

Rabelais calls this "blasphemy." The prophet who announced what is false and harmful is not a prophet of the Lord, but a prophet of the Devil. False prophets are demonic men and women, in the service of untruth and darkness. To blame God and the servants of God (saints, angels, and so on) for the evils of the world is to imagine the divine in the image of the worst, most petulant sort of humankind. Is it pious to blame all human suffering on the cruelty of a vengeful god? Is it love of God that leads us to attribute natural disasters and pestilences to divine retaliation? Is it holy to believe that the malice of an outraged divinity can be bribed and placated by prayer? Those religious authorities and faith leaders who announce such things turn the masses away from the love of God. One may fear and obey a despot who rules with arbitrary power, but one does not love such a lord. To turn away from the divine in this manner is to turn toward the kingdom of darkness.

This is the message implicit in Rabelais. False prophets of divine vengeance "poison souls." They work against enlightenment, which is the necessary basis of real medical progress and the establishment of human precautions against plague and other disasters. The idea that "only a God can save us" leads to humiliation and obedient quietism. It keeps the

---

9 John L. Micek, "In resolution, Pa. lawmaker blames COVID-19 outbreak on 'our presumptuous sins,'" *The Philadelphia Tribune* (24 Mar. 2020).

masses enthralled to religious authority and unaware of their own potentialities. The belief that humans can save other humans through knowledge and action is a principle of Renaissance humanism. *Homo homini Deus est.* Rabelais the physician, the student of the new methods of observation and experimentation, sees the superstition taught by false ministers as a spiritual poison just as harmful as the bodily poison of disease.

Grandgousier is, for Rabelais, the paradigm of a good king in many ways. His action against the "false prophet" in his kingdom is swift and severe, and sends a message to all future pretenders. This is Rabelais' suggestion for how secular power ought always to behave toward pernicious zealotry. The poisoner of souls should be punished more severely than the poisoner of bodies. The latter can take a few lives at most, but the former debases the inner life of whole congregations at a time. The knave Panurge spreads plague with his fecal concoction, and we can laugh at this because we see in this action the absurdity of human folly. Panurge is a trickster, but the trickster is an important figure. Trickster divinities (Hermes, Pan, Prometheus) are responsible for making the human world, bringing light to the darkness.[10] Religious fear, on the other hand, is pathetic, and *pathos* in its original sense means "disease." Fear, like pity or rage, is *pathos* because it is an affliction that comes from without, over which the subject has no control. It is no less contagious than fever. The spreading of spiritual poison is not comic, but demonic, and the false prophet destroys the human world, bringing darkness to the light.

Grandgousier gives the pilgrims counsel concerning what they ought to be doing instead of prostrating themselves before the shrine of the saint. He says, "Go your way, poor folk, in the name of God the Creator; may He be a perpetual guide to you, and henceforth don't be easy marks for those otiose and useless trips. Look after your families, each man work in his vocation, bring up your children, and live as the good Apostle Saint Paul teaches you to do. So doing, you will have the protection of God, the angels, and the saints with you, and there will be neither plague nor trouble that will do you harm!" (104–5). The "easy mark" is not guiltless; assent or dissent is always within one's power. The pilgrims recognize the wisdom of this advice, and praise the sagacity of the king to Gargantua: "We are more edified and instructed by these words than by all the sermons ever preached to us in our town" (105). Rabelais here inserts a reflection on the

---

10 See Lewis Hyde, *Trickster Makes this World* (New York: Farras, Straus & Giroux, 1988).

justice of Plato's doctrine of the philosopher king.[11]

Rabelais teaches that these pilgrimages and actions that are aimed at bribing and appeasing the saints and the gods are so much wasted energy. Apart from their futility, these pilgrimages are dangerous and actively pernicious, being conducive to the spread of the contagion and the worsening of conditions. Bands of poor, downtrodden peasants roam from town to town, interacting with locals for their sustenance, and sleeping where they can along their route. These are the conditions under which contagion is promiscuously spread. Instead of such harmful adventures in piety, Rabelais asserts that one's time would be much better spent staying at home, doing one's work, living an upright life, and caring for one's family and property. If God is to be "placated," it is only by tending conscientiously to the fruits of the world. To live in this way, and to lay aside unreasonable fears and superstitions, is the best way to preserve oneself and win the protection of the heavens. To waste one's powers by journeying to pay respects to all of the shrines of Europe is to amuse only the devils of this world and to ignore those activities for which human beings are made.

This doctrine has much in common with the classical doctrine of the Stoics concerning those things that are in one's control and those things that are not. It is fully within our power to determine what we do, how we handle our business, what we eat, and with whom we interact. Since these things depend entirely on our judgment and the use we make of impressions, we ought to proceed with due caution and care in making our decisions. External things are less susceptible to our control. Plague is an external thing, and its spread is something that does not depend on our will. Therefore, it is proper to adopt an attitude of confidence toward plague and other diseases, knowing that if they come they come, through no fault of our own. Dread is wasted on those hazards that are beyond our power. Continuing to lead a good life, a life of integrity, is the best response to pandemics.[12] Stoicism is always a sound doctrine when times are lean, just as Epicureanism is sound when times are fat.

In spite of his ridicule of misguided religious authorities, Rabelais is not an opponent of religion. Renaissance humanism is opposed to superstition, though it is a mistake to believe that humanism is opposed to religion in general. The Renaissance is sometimes incorrectly thought of as a

11 See Plato, *Rep.* V: "Until philosophers rule as kings or those who are now called kings and leading men genuinely and adequately philosophize, that is, until political power and philosophy entirely coincide … cities will have no rest from evils, Glaucon, nor, I think, will the human race" (473c–d).

12 See, for instance, Epictetus, *Discourses*, II.i.

mere prelude to the atheism or deism characteristic of the Enlightenment *philosophes* of two hundred years later. This is a misunderstanding. Many Renaissance thinkers were concerned with reforming the abuses of the Church, but would have balked at the idea of undermining religious sentiment writ large. The Protestant Reformation is not a radical break from earlier Renaissance thought, but a continuation of many of its guiding ideas. The Renaissance scholar Paul Oskar Kristeller asserts with plausibility that there were very few real atheists during the Renaissance. He writes, "If an age where the nonreligious concerns that had been growing for centuries attained a kind of equilibrium with religious and theological thought, or even began to surpass it in vitality and appeal, must be called pagan, the Renaissance was pagan, at least in certain places and phases. Yet since the religious convictions of Christianity were either retained or transformed, but never really challenged, it seems more appropriate to call the Renaissance a fundamentally Christian age."[13]

Rabelais was himself a priest and monk, belonging first to the strict Observantine Franciscan order, and later residing in Benedictine monasteries. He was the friend and client of bishop and popes. He did father several illegitimate children as a priest, but they were legitimized by papal decree, and though he became a secular priest later in life, it was only because the abbey to which he was attached was secularized. There is no reason to doubt his religious convictions as a Christian. He saw the Pyrrhonian skepticism that had been recently rediscovered as silly: "Truly from now on it will be possible to catch lions by the thick hair, horses by the mane, oxen by the horns, wild oxen by the muzzle, wolves by the tail, goats by the beard, birds by the feet; but never will such [Pyrrhonian] philosophers be caught by their words" (367–68).[14]

This religious conviction makes Rabelais' criticism of "false prophets" all the more damning. Religion itself is not at fault; religion is a consolation in times of suffering and a reservoir of psychological fortitude. It is the men—or devils—who preach falsely that compromise the soul of the believer and the well-being of the community. These men take advantage of their positions of authority and spread untruths. These untruths stoke the religious dread of the masses, and this fear before the divine disables the faculty of reason. As Vico says, the thunder of Jove humbles the bodies

13 Paul Oskar Kristeller, *Renaissance Thought* (New York: Harper & Row, 1961), 73.

14 Richard Popkin calls this passage "the most famous discussion of Pyrrhonism in [the Renaissance]." *The History of Skepticism: From Savonarola to Bayle* (New York: Oxford University Press, 2003), 27–28.

and minds of humans.[15] Men and women are persuaded to adopt counter-productive modes of behavior and fail to recognize the true nature of the threat of plague. Rather than tending to their business and families, they are sent on fantastic quests far from home to placate the bones of saints. They carry contagion with them, or pick it up along the route. At the same time, the affairs of the hearth are left to ruin. Rabelais is sincere in his assertion that real piety consists of minding one's business.

Rabelais' authority is that of both cleric and physician. He knows that the transmission of contagion has natural causes. There are worldly phenomena that explain infection, and no appeal to divine retaliation is needed. Human beings cannot feel themselves to be disapproved of by the divine without trembling. The great power of the Hebrew prophets is causing sinners to tremble, but in their case the reason for this is to compel moral changes that are within human power. In the case of pandemics, religious panic keeps us from seeing clearly what steps are necessary to confront a crisis born of this world. Observation teaches that plague *does not* spare the righteous and claim the guilty. It *does* spare the solitary and claim the promiscuous. The human obtuseness that fails to learn the clear lessons of experience always has an aura of the comical and absurd. We may laugh with Rabelais at the pious pilgrims who do not recognize their own folly. However, he also teaches us a serious lesson that remains relevant today: keep rational, do not give in to panic, and continue in your station.

15 Vico, *New Science*, §502.

CHAPTER V

Daniel Defoe

A Journal of the Plague Year

Quarantine is the Mandate of Wisdom

In 1720, London was seriously threatened by plague for the first time in half a century. Bubonic plague arrived in Marseilles from Asia, and within a few months had taken 40,000 French lives. English sentiment was mixed. Because of the significance of Marseilles as a major hub of maritime trade, an outbreak on English soil was seen as a real possibility by many persons in positions of authority. Physicians composed or reissued treatises on public health and the government took legislative steps to prevent a visitation of the Black Death, such as the enforcement of mandatory quarantine for all ships arriving from infected regions. However, the public was skeptical about the reality of the threat, and the unpopularity of many of the preventative measures taken by the government led to much public derision. Novel restrictions on personal freedom are always met with resistance when they are enacted, in the absence of a clear *immediate* danger. Administrative and popular opinion stood in open conflict regarding the severity of the threat of a new outbreak. Many accused the crown of tyrannical overreach, and others, like the future bishop of London, Edmund Gibson, defended the necessity of severe measures: "Where the disease is desperate, the Remedy must be so too; and to dwell upon *Rights* and *Liberties* ... is as wild a Way of Reasoning, as if under a malignant Fever we should insist on being dealt with in all respects like Men in perfect Health."[1]

This mixed response is indicative of a tendency for collective repression of trauma and evidence for William James' doctrine that forgetting is just as necessary for psychological health as memory.[2] In 1665, London had been devastated by the Great Plague, which had caused the death of a quarter of the city's population, roughly 100,000 souls. Nevertheless, five decades later, its denizens were willing to hazard the same bleak conditions for the sake of their liberty of movement and association.

---

1 See Charles F. Mullett, "The English plague scare of 1720–23," *Osiris* 2 (1936): 484–516 (Gibson qtd. at 492).

2 William James, *Principles of Psychology* (New York: Dover, 1950), I:679–80.

Daniel Defoe (1660–1731), best known today for his novels *Robinson Crusoe* and *Moll Flanders*, wrote *A Journal of the Plague Year* within the context of this social situation. The narrative is ostensibly a firsthand account of London during the Great Plague of 1665. Defoe was himself five years old at the time, so its "author" is credited as "H. F." (probably a reference to Defoe's uncle, Henry Foe, whose biography shares much with the story's narrator). The book is an exemplary work of historical fiction, copiously researched and interspersed with statistical tables. Defoe's intention in composing the book is twofold: both to alert the English public to the horrors of the plague, and to consider what measures—both public and private—are most effective in meliorating its harm, and which are counter-productive. The *Journal* is in accord with the progressive idea of its time that social leaders could work to *prevent* pathological outbreaks rather than merely offering medical intervention to those already infected.[3] To that end, it is a largely didactic in tone.

What we learn from Defoe's *Journal* is the fundamental importance of avoiding public space during a pandemic. The only way one can stay entirely safe from infection is altogether to avoid physical contact with other persons, or to flee from an area at the first rumor of infection. Likewise, infected persons must be isolated from others to prevent their spreading the disease by contact. It would be nearly two centuries before the *Y. pestis* bacterium was identified and the causes of the spread of plague were fully understood. Nevertheless, prudence and experience taught the educated European of the time that transmission was the result of proximity to the infected, and not the work of occult or divine forces.

The Lord Mayor of London published an order in 1665 that, "As soon as any man shall be found by [a public] examiner, chirurgeon, or searcher to be sick of the plague, he shall the same night be sequestered in the same house; and in case he be so sequestered, then, though he afterwards die not, the house wherein he sickened should be shut up for a month, the use of the due preservatives taken by the rest." (48).[4] Other orders commanded that any person having contact with an infected person was "shut up for certain days by the examiner's discretion"; persons sharing a house where infection was known to have struck were not to remove from that house without permission from a medical examiner; no furniture or other material things were to be removed from infected houses; and

3 See Mullett, "Plague scare," 486.

4 All parenthetical citations in this section refer to Daniel Defoe, *A Journal of the Plague Year* (New York: Signet, 1960).

infected houses were to be clearly marked with a red cross, locked up, and monitored by constables (48–51). These orders show that the London political administration was convinced that quarantining infected persons was of the utmost importance for curtailing the speed with which the plague was transmitted.

There is no doubt that isolating those who carry infection is a necessary public health measure. However, quarantining only the sick is an *ipso facto* measure that comes too late, and condemning all members of the household to share in the quarantine of an infected person is Draconian. Defoe's first insight is that the most effective prevention of the spread of disease is universal preemptive quarantine. Asymptomatic carriers are far more likely to transmit plague than those visibly in its throes, whom others know to avoid. If quarantine is imposed only on those who are demonstrably ill, then the damage of mass transmission has already been wrought. The public must be educated in the need for isolation even among persons in robust health.

Defoe's second insight is that such quarantine must be self-imposed rather than mandated by authority. Human beings may or may not be "social animals" by nature, but they are certainly made so by habit. They are also disinclined to wager with death by remaining in a residence where there is a known infection. The compulsory power of any legal mandate comes from the threat of force that underlies the order. The individual performs a practical calculus when considering whether to obey a given law. He or she weighs the potential cost of transgression against the certain cost of submission. In order to totally overcome the sociable habits and instincts of self-preservation shared by all civilized humans, a quarantine law would have to threaten the most extreme violence to transgressors. If such severe measures are necessary in order to preserve a polity, perhaps that polity is not worth preserving. As Cicero observes, "There are some acts either so repulsive or so wicked, that a wise man would not commit them, even to save his country. … The wise man, therefore, will not think of doing any such thing for the sake of his country; no more will his country consent to have it done for her."[5] It is not law that must compel quarantine; it is sympathy and understanding both one's own interests and the interests of society.

This does not mean that compulsory quarantine was altogether a misstep on the part of officials. There was a clear and present need for shutting

---

5 Cicero, *On Duties*, trans. Walter Miller (Cambridge, MA: Harvard University Press, 1913), I.xlv.159.

up "the distempered people, who would otherwise have been both very troublesome and very dangerous in their running about streets with the distemper on them" (159). Had the sick not been confined, "multitudes who, in the height of their fever, were delirious and distracted would have been continually running up and down the streets; and even as it was a very great number did so" (161). Defoe is not opposed to forced quarantine, but he found its implementation misdirected.

In spite of the statutes passed by London's Lord Mayor, Defoe says, "Many such escapes were made out of infected houses. … People got two or three keys made to their locks, or they found ways to unscrew the locks such as were screwed on" (57). Others employed more elaborate and inventive means of escaping from infected houses, which were effectively "prisons without bars" (59). If signs of plague were noted in a servant, whole families would stealthily retreat from the home before alerting the authorities. More conscientious families that did stay in place would predictably spread the infection one to another, and entire households would be killed where many could have been preserved. Some persons were overcome with the madness brought on by mortal terror and ran manically through the streets, spreading infection. Others refused to acknowledge their own symptoms and unwittingly served as ravagers. Defoe writes, "Those that did thus break out spread the infection farther by their wandering about with the distemper on them, in their desperate circumstances, than they would otherwise have done" (60).

Legal mandates alone—regardless of the severity of the penalties for transgression—were unable to compel quarantine. Defoe observes, "The severities that were used, though grievous in themselves, had also this further objection against them, namely, that they did not answer the end, as I have said, but that the distempered people went day by day about the streets" (168). A law that fails to answer its own end is not only useless, but actively pernicious to the respect that citizens ought to feel for law in general.

Defoe's counsel is to isolate infected persons from the rest of their households, rather than condemning entire families to exposure. Such a "demi-quarantine" requires foresight, as designated houses and institutions must be established for the isolation of the sound. Defoe argues that "if houses had been provided on purpose for those that were sound to perform this demi-quarantine in, they would have much less reason to think themselves injured in such a restraint than in being confined with infected people in the houses where they lived" (169). This separation of the sick from the well is demanded by basic humanity. In the modern world, hospitals and other institutions exist that fill this role, though they are presently taxed beyond their limits by COVID-19 and are often unable to provide quarantine to the extent demanded by the crisis.

The shortcomings of the London statutes regarding isolation are a secondary issue for confronting the plague. This relates us back to Defoe's first insight, that quarantining only those already visibly infected or exposed to infection is an insufficient measure, even if its execution could be perfected. Proactive quarantine is needed for prevention of infection. Defoe writes, "Nothing was more fatal to the inhabitants of this city than the supine negligence of the people themselves, who, during the long notice or warning they had of the visitation, made no provision for it, by laying in store of provisions, or of other necessaries, by which they might have lived retired, and within their own houses, as I have observed others did, and who were in a great measure preserved by that caution" (80). Material needs compelled healthy persons to enter the marketplace, and this intermingling in public space for the acquisition of provisions "was in a great measure the ruin of the whole city" (82).

Pandemics are so difficult to fight because the enemy is invisible. Every human being with rudimentary observational faculties has the prudence to avoid contact with symptomatic persons. However, overt signs of infection are typically inscribed on the body and behavior of the sick only in the later developments of the disease. Pandemic diseases are infectious prior to the onset of such overt symptoms.[6] The line between "sick" and "well" is equivocal. Infectious disease cannot be thought of in a binary manner with the line drawn at the presentation of symptoms (this person is "sick" because she manifests these symptoms, this person is "well" because he does not). Those who are to all appearances "well" may very well carry the seeds of illness about with them. Such persons bear the character of the mower in the old German hymn: "There is a mower death yclept. Hath power that the lord hath kept. When he begins his scythe to whet, keener it grows and keener yet."[7]

Defoe writes, "It was not the sick people only from whom the plague was immediately received by others that were sound, but the well. To explain myself, by the sick people I mean those who were known to be sick

6 This was obvious three centuries ago, but is news to political leaders today. Georgia governor Brian Kemp, for instance, claimed to have learned this only on 1 April, 2020, a month into the COVID-19 outbreak in America.

7 I am unable to discover the original source of this hymn. It appears repeatedly in the novel *Berlin Alexanderplatz* by Alfred Döblin.

... these everybody could beware of; they were either in their beds or in such condition as could not be concealed. By the well I mean such as had received the contagion, and had it really upon them, and in their blood, yet did not show the consequences of it in their countenances; nay, even were not sensible of it themselves" (187). These asymptomatic carriers are the people most dangerous to others, through no fault of their own. "These were the people of whom the well people ought to have been afraid; but then, on the other side, it was impossible to know them. And this is the reason why it is impossible in a visitation to prevent the spreading of the plague by the utmost human vigilance, viz., that it is impossible to know the infected people from the sound, or that the infected people should perfectly know themselves" (188).

The most tragic aspect of this invisibility of the bacterium is its consequence for intimate contact. Lover infects the beloved, parent infects child. Filial and erotic love terminate in the same result as malice or cruelty. Defoe writes, "It was very sad to reflect how such a person ... had ruined those that he would have hazarded his life to save, and had been breathing death upon them, even perhaps in his tender kissing and embracings of his children." We must ask with resignation, "If then the blow is thus insensibly striking, if the arrow flies thus unseen, and cannot be discovered, to what purpose are all the schemes for shutting up or removing the sick people?" (198). This presents a serious dilemma for the philosopher. The rules of moral behavior, which should be universal and unchanging, must undergo a revaluation in times of crisis. Love demands withdrawal and renunciation, attraction demands repulsion. In this situation, the temptation to be avoided is the behavior that morality commands under average circumstances. The "good" is the temptation, as it is in the paradoxes of Søren Kierkegaard.[8] An inverted moral world is established, like that described by Hegel: "What in the law of the first is sweet, in this inverted in-itself is sour, what in the former is black is, in the other, white."[9] We have only prudence to guide us between Scylla and Charybdis.

These considerations remain pressingly relevant to our situation today. While officials in China and other nations have acted swiftly and decisively, American politicians on both the federal and local levels have

---

8 See Kierkegaard's analysis of the paradoxical moral situation in the story of Abraham and Isaac from Gen. 22, "a paradox that makes a murder into a holy and God-pleasing act." *Fear and Trembling*, trans. Howard V. Hong and Edna H. Hong (Princeton, NJ: Princeton University Press, 1983), 53.

9 G. W. F. Hegel, *Phenomenology of Spirit*, trans. A. V. Miller (New York: Oxford University Press, 1977), §158.

made a concerted effort to avoid definitive statements or actions concerning the scope of shelter-in-place orders and the level to which quarantine will be enforced, leaving such things to the arbitrary will of local law enforcement. This is tactful; negative public response to government mandates in London in both 1665 and 1720 demonstrate the political expedience of non-action. However, it is also socially harmful. Leadership is needed in times of crisis, but the modern democratic politician avoids taking any position. What is needed are "statesmen," persons gifted in prudence with the courage to apply wisdom to action. The politician today is a master of the techniques of self-preservation and self-promotion, but lacks the virtue of statecraft. Skill in amassing votes is not the same as skill in leadership.

Defoe shows us the best route to safety. He writes, "A vast number of people locked themselves up, so as not to come abroad into any company at all, nor suffer any that had been abroad in promiscuous company to come into their houses, or near them." Public space was not hazarded and necessary intercourse with strangers was carried out at a distance. "When people began to use these cautions they were less exposed to danger, and the infection did not break into such houses so furiously as it did into others before; and thousands of families were preserved, speaking with due reserve to the direction of Divine Providence, by that means" (204–5). This attitude was late in arising, and was by no means universal, with greater numbers adopting a melancholy resignation to predestined fate. However, the majority of those who did adopt an isolationist attitude and understood the necessity of limiting contact with the outside world were by and large preserved.

Defoe teaches that careful quarantine is the best preservative of life and health. The counsel of Defoe is sound for all times: *plague conditions require a disciplined quarantine maintained by wisdom, not compulsion.* Foresight is necessary when plague conditions threaten; prevention is more imperative and more successful than treatment. This means that provisions must be amassed, and conscientious people must be prepared for an extended period of spatial solitude. However, compulsory isolation is both ineffective and inhumane. Even the visibly infected cannot be restrained in place if they fail to internalize the reasons behind this imperative. The citizens of London only discovered the need for self-quarantine through much experience of the ravages of promiscuous sociability. Harsh reality brought them to will quarantine for themselves. Defoe intended the Londoners of the 1720s to be taught by the suffering of their progenitors of 1665. We may absorb this lesson as well, and take the *Journal* as a guidebook for cautious behavior.

To be effective, the law of quarantine must be given to oneself. This is the meaning of "autonomy": self-ruling, giving oneself the law. Autonomy is not unbridled license, but the self-generation of rules of behavior. This is the only kind of true freedom that there is. Lawless license is not freedom, but bondage to the passions. Autonomous behavior overcomes passion through self-control. Wisdom itself counsels quarantine, and to obey this dictum is to demonstrate one's mastery over all passionate impulses. The establishment for oneself of a prison without bars is paradoxically required in the name of freedom.

Quarantine is much less impactful for us than it was for our ancestors. *Robinson Crusoe* is the novel of the isolated man, and one would need to be another Crusoe to live outside of the public sphere in the eighteenth century. Such total isolation is the "Island of Despair."[10] This is no longer the case. Quarantine is certainly still a vexation. Every situation that dams up the regular flow of one's life is a nuisance that requires a stoical attitude and time for adaptation. However, the human being is an infinitely adaptable creature. Juan Luis Vives' fable about man tells us that, "As he of gods the greatest, embracing all things in his might, is all things, they saw man, Jupiter's mime, be all things also."[11] Quarantine is less pernicious today than it was for previous generations because of the mediation of technology. To be rooted in place is no longer a condemnation to social exile. There is very little social behavior that cannot be fabricated virtually. Friends are no more distant, conversation no less accessible. Museums can be toured, concerts attended, romances kindled, all in the virtual realm of cyberspace. To mistake technologically mediated activity with authentic human action is a mistake. I have argued elsewhere against the seductions of technology and the idolization of this form of "hyperreality."[12] However, when properly understood as fabrication and used as an instrument in the service of humanistic ends, modern technology is superlatively useful.

There is a deeper issue than mere spatial isolation. Everyday life under reasonably healthful conditions has its own patterns and regularity. This regularity is comforting and psychologically edifying. We feel that

---

10 Daniel Defoe, *Robinson Crusoe* (New York: Bantam, 1981), 61.

11 Juan Luis Vives, "A Fable about Man," trans. Nancy Lenkeith, in *The Renaissance Philosophy of Man*, ed. Ernst Cassirer, Paul Oskar Kristeller, and John Herman Randall, Jr. (Chicago: University of Chicago Press, 1948), 389.

12 See my *Shame, Fame, and the Technological Mentality*, chap. 3.

we understand the rules of the various social "games" that we play, and we understand our place within the context of the various groups to which we belong. In times of crisis, whether the crisis is medical, military, economic, or otherwise, this regularity is compromised. We experience what the sociologist Émile Durkheim calls "anomy," that is, the upheaval of social order and the breakdown of traditional regulations and standards of comportment. Durkheim writes, "So long as the social forces thus freed have not regained equilibrium, their respective values are unknown and so all regulation is lacking for a time. The limits are unknown between the possible and the impossible, what is just and what is unjust, legitimate claims and hopes and those which are immoderate. Consequently, there is no restraint upon aspirations."[13] We feel ourselves thrown off balance, cast into a foreign reality, strangers in our own land. We no longer understand how things are ordered, or where to look for orientation. The games of human life suddenly change their rules.

When large-scale breaks in continuity occur, it becomes necessary to establish new modes of regularity. Plagues carry chaos in their wake, but they also bring about new orderly formations of the world. This phenomenon has been described by Michel Foucault. He writes, "The plague is met by order; its function is to sort out every possible confusion: that of the disease, which is transmitted when bodies are mixed together; that of the evil which is increased when fear and death overcome prohibitions. It lays down for each individual his place, his body, his disease, and his death ... even to the ultimate determination of the individual, of what characterizes him, of what belongs to him, of what happens to him. Against the plague, which is a mixture, discipline brings into play its power, which is one of analysis."[14] Outbreaks of plague produce anomic conditions, which psycho-social needs compel human beings to attempt to obviate. While it is common for literature to reflect the bacchic festival of anomy that characterizes the early stages of an outbreak, Foucault highlights "a political dream of the plague, which was exactly its reverse: not the collective festival, but strict divisions; not laws transgressed, but the penetration of regulation into even the smallest details of everyday life through the mediation of the complete hierarchy that assured the capillary functioning of power; not masks that were put on and off, but the assignment to each

---

13 Émile Durkheim, *Suicide*, trans. John A Spaulding and George Simpson (New York: Free Press, 1979), 253. See the whole of Bk. 2, chap. 5, "Anomic Suicide."

14 Michel Foucault, *Discipline and Punish*, trans. Alan Sheridan (New York: Vintage, 1995), 197.

individual of his 'true' name, his 'true' place, his 'true' body, his 'true' disease. The plague as a form, at once real and imaginary, of disorder had as its medical and political correlative *discipline*."[15]

This movement from anomic conditions—the chaotic herd madness of failed social institutions—to new modes of discipline and regulation is illustrated in the drama of Defoe's *Journal*. From the very start of plague conditions in London, local administration attempts to impose regularity with comprehensive orders for the social sphere. New magistracies and offices are established with the responsibility of overseeing and enforcing these orders. Statutes are even promulgated regulating the permissible behavior of "loose persons and idle assemblies," like beggars, stage actors, and drinking establishments (52–53). The same discipline is imposed upon these fringe elements of society, which are characterized by their general disorder, as the middle class and the bourgeoisie. The discipline legislated under these circumstances is far more severe than that of "normal" times. Foucault writes, "In order to see perfect disciplines functioning, rulers dreamt of the state of plague. Underlying disciplinary projects the image of the plague stands for all forms of confusion and disorder."[16] London saw such projects implemented in 1665.

However, we have already seen that legislative regulation by itself is ineffective, and that the hyper-disciplinary statutes of the London government failed on their own to impose good order and regulated behavior. It is only the internalization of the principles of discipline that led to substantive change and melioration of the pandemic. The lesson to be learned from this is that government intervention can only go so far toward establishing new modes of regulation and discipline. Externally imposed quarantine and other extreme and unusual methods of order are insufficient. So long as such commands are seen as impersonal, oppressive, and unnecessary, they are felt to be acts of violence rather than acts of benevolence. The equivocal language and mixed messaging of politicians only inflames this suspicion. The good effects of these legal commands must be understood by the individual members of society in order for the necessary social discipline to take hold.

This was the hard lesson learned in 1665 through gruesome experience. This is the lesson that Defoe intended to impart a half century later during the next London plague scare. The same truths hold for us today. If we would learn this lesson with minimal personal suffering, we must cast

15 Ibid., 197–98, emphasis added.
16 Ibid., 199.

ourselves into the *Journal*'s narrative, and experience the tragedy of that age with sympathy, not as scenes from a dead world, but as a moving gallery of images alive to us today. When history reveals patterns, taking the past as a tutorial is the surest way to combat its repetition. The people of London were preserved when they stopped entering public space and took real precautions in their dealings with others. This is a difficult lesson to learn, and harder still to take on authority, but, as Defoe says, "A plague is a formidable enemy, and is armed with terrors that every man is not sufficiently fortified to resist or prepared to stand the shock against" (229). Confronting such a formidable enemy requires much sacrifice and radically new social forms.

The upheaval of one's life in times of plague is traumatic, but this trauma can be mollified. The psychological harm of any large-scale crisis is largely a result of the experience of anomy, the breakdown of traditional regulatory principles. Rediscovering equilibrium and steady ground requires developing new norms of behavior. New rules of discipline must come from within. This self-discipline, or self-control, is the best means to ensure prevention of infection. The important work of every individual must be to develop new modes of personal behavior and new patterns of life that reintroduce regularity and order. The choice of these modes is autonomous, and must be so. The rule of life must be given by oneself to oneself. The agent may then take pride in having benefitted both himself and society as a whole.

The severe discipline required by the need for quarantine is therefore a work of moral cultivation. It entails engagement with questions about the nature of the good life. Legal prohibitions can go so far as to overturn the old way of life, but it is only humane philosophy that can establish new ways. Jurisprudence builds and sustains nations. Culture, on the other hand, is not born of jurisprudence, but of human leisure and contemplation.[17] Quarantine is not an absolute evil, and like all other existential realities, we learn to adapt to its exigency. But to do so, we must first impose it as a law on ourselves, and then establish new patterns of activity and behavior. This is a practice in discipline of the self by the self.

---

17 See Josef Pieper, *Leisure, the Basis of Culture*, trans. Gerald Malsbary (South Bend, IN: St. Augustine Press, 1998).

CHAPTER VI

Alessandro Manzoni

The Betrothed

Forgive Enemies and Evolve

The Great Plague of Milan was a series of outbreaks of bubonic plague that scourged northern and central Italy between the years 1629 and 1631. During this pandemic, mortality rates in these regions were higher than they had been during any occurrence of plague since the Black Death three centuries earlier. Of 130,000 people then living in Milan, a minimum of 60,000 lost their lives to the outbreak. Other cities fared just as poorly; over sixty percent of the population of Verona died during that time, and Venice lost 46,000 souls. In the whole of northern Italy, around a million people died, a quarter of the entire regional population. Another million persons likely fell ill, but survived the pandemic. This catastrophe fortunately marked the last outbreak of plague for most of the cities of the area.[1]

The effect of large-scale disasters on major social institutions is often the subject of scholarly research. Historians grapple with questions about the extent to which the Black Death helped to shape the early Italian Renaissance or the Thirty Years' War led to the new political model of sovereign nation-states. Any major catastrophe marks an abrupt break in the continuity of a civilization. It sharply reveals the deficiencies in the reigning status quo, and recovery from catastrophe usually requires the adoption of new social forms. After they initially come into being, nations strive for regularity and order. This is necessary for tranquility and economic stability, but the negative aspect of this phenomenon is a corresponding tendency for cultural petrification. The longer a nation's way of life has persisted, the more ingrained are its distinctive ideas and prejudices. Technologies may progress with astounding rapidity, but culture on the whole remains stagnant. Once petrification has set in, it is often only a major, unforeseen epochal event that can shake the character of the nation. Major national wars, natural disasters, and serious epidemics are all evils that one ought never to desire. However, very few things are altogether without

1 These statistics are taken from J. N. Hays, *Epidemics and Pandemics: Their Impacts on Human History* (Santa Barbara, CA: ABC-Clio, 2005), 103.

benefit. Such disasters can often reenergize a stagnant people and invigorate human ingenuity. Social life is compelled to adopt new organizations, which carry culture forward.

Every political scientist is aware of the destructive-creative impact of cataclysm on societies. Political scientists ignore, however, a parallel phenomenon that occurs on the level of the particular human being. Sociologists explore the effect of circumstances on particular humans, but always in the abstract, as faceless statistics. The impact of major disasters on the concrete *individual*—as is true of all things at the individual level—is the province of literature and the other humanities.

Just as the course of nations and societies suffers interruption and reorganization as consequences of disasters, so does the individual human life. Human character often appears unruly and protean as it manifests itself. Nevertheless, it is usually possible in hindsight to discover a reasonably stable trajectory of an individual's life. This was the insight of Jean-Paul Sartre's doctrine of "existential psychoanalysis." Sartre writes, "The being considered does not crumble into dust, and one can discover in him that unity … which must be a unity of responsibility, a unity of agreeable or hateful, blamable and praiseworthy, in short *personal*. This unity, which is the being of the man under consideration, is a *free unification*, and this unification cannot come *after* a diversity which it unifies."[2] An individual tends to organize his or her life in reference to certain principles of behavior and certain regular fields of activity. One's personal history is fairly linear. A handful of foundational ideas inform one's actions, pursuits, and emotions. A few projects of personal ambition are prioritized, and life unfurls as the pursuit of these goals. As external circumstances change, the manner of this pursuit alters, but the goals themselves and the foundational ideas on which they are built remain relatively stable. This produces a unity, which is called one's integral character. We could also call it one's *style*.

Under stable conditions, there is no impetus for this integral character to change. Crisis situations can, however, interrupt the linear development of the individual and reorder one's foundational ideas and principles. This is part of the reason soldiers often have difficulty reassimilating to peacetime society and trauma survivors struggle with idle chatter. We often see such phenomena occur in literary works, particularly with respect to the disruptive power of war. The general flow of a character's

2 Jean-Paul Sartre, *Being and Nothingness*, trans. Hazel E. Barnes (New York: Washington Square Press, 1984), 717.

development proceeds along a more or less linear path. Represented graphically, there are peaks and valleys, but the line consistently moves in the same direction. This is the mythical cord of life spun and manipulated by the Fates. The sudden onset of war is like a perpendicular line that severs this natural flow. When we meet our characters again after this crisis, their situations are upset, their values reordered, and a new set of objectives gives meaning and style to their lives.

Thomas Mann's *The Magic Mountain* is such a book. The drama of the vast majority of the novel concerns the minutiae of life at a sanatorium. We watch the characters slowly develop relationships with one another, their psychologies are laboriously scrutinized, and as readers we become deeply invested in the day-to-day temperature readings and minor complaints of the half-sick population. Suddenly, and without warning, the narrative is abruptly cut through by the outbreak of the Great War. The final chapter is aptly titled "The Thunderbolt." The thunderbolt announces the presence of new gods and the death of the old world. In Vico's *New Science*, the thunderbolt "humbled not only their bodies but their minds as well, by creating in [primitive humans] this frightful idea of Jove."[3] The new idea of Jove introduces a new morality into the world. The same is true of the bombing raids of World War I, that "historic thunder-peal, of which we speak with bated breath, [which] made the foundations of the earth to shake."[4] New gods, new moralities, and new modes of existence emerge by necessity. Suddenly, our hero, Hans Castorp, is thrown into the theater of war, running through the mud, possibly hit by enemy fire, perhaps alive, perhaps dead. We then lose sight of him altogether, and the story is over. Mann writes, "Shame on our shadow-safety! Away! No more!"[5]

Marcel Proust's *In Search of Lost Time* is another novel that is suddenly and violently interrupted by the same war. Six volumes develop with a meticulous slowness, the scenes of the narrator's adolescence painted with pain-staking detail. The book's cyclical patterns of emotion and behavior work themselves out in ever-larger spirals. Time itself becomes a central subject of the novel, as it is for Proust's cousin-by-marriage, Henri Bergson. Pages and pages, thousands of words, are devoted to the recollection of a *petite madeleine* eaten once long ago. Suddenly, in the seventh

3 Vico, *New Science*, §502.
4 Thomas Mann, *The Magic Mountain*, trans. H. T. Lowe-Porter (New York: Alfred A. Knopf, 1946), 709.
5 Ibid., 715.

volume, the war erupts, and the continuity of the past is interrupted. The war is the dramatic break in which time is lost. We are reunited with our characters after the war, but all relationships are altered, all priorities are now different. "'Trees,' thought I to myself, 'you have nothing more to say to me; my deadened heart no longer hears you. ... If there was once a time when I was able to believe myself a poet, I now know that I am not. In the new chapter of my now arid life which is opening before me, perhaps men might be able to give me the inspiration I no longer find in nature. But the days when I might possibly have been able to sing her praises will return no more.'"[6] The people on whom the narrator once built his life are barely recognized when he meets them again.

Plague may have the same effect on character and style as war. The great novel in which this is the case is *The Betrothed* (*I promessi sposi*), written by Alessandro Manzoni (1785–1873) in 1823–27. *The Betrothed* is the most widely-read of all Italian novels, and Daniel Burt has claimed that "no other work in Italy other than Dante's *Divine Comedy* has done more to establish the literary language of Italian."[7] Umberto Eco (who adapted *The Betrothed* into an illustrated novel for a younger audience) once wrote, "Almost all Italians hate [*The Betrothed*] because they were forced to read it in school. My father, however, encouraged me to read *I promessi sposi* before my teachers forced me to, and I love it."[8] The majority of *The Betrothed* is a pastoral romance, in which unfortunate young lovers strive to be united despite forces hostile to their union. The Great Plague of Milan is the perpendicular catastrophe that suddenly interrupts the narrative and reorganizes the lives of heroes and antagonists alike.

Manzoni was himself Milanese, descended from feudal lords, and the grandson of the philosopher Cesare Beccaria, best known for his treatise *On Crimes and Punishments*. Along with Sir Walter Scott, Manzoni was one of the earliest European masters of the historical novel. In his influential essay *On the Historical Novel*, he writes, "The principle subject of the historical novel is completely the author's, completely poetic, because merely verisimilar. Both the purpose and design of the author are, as much as possible, to make the subject and all the action so verisimilar with

6 Marcel Proust, *The Past Recaptured*, in *Remembrance of Things Past*, trans. C. K. Scott Moncrieff and Frederick A. Blossom (New York: Random House, 1932), II:983.

7 Daniel S. Burt, *The Novel 100* (New York: Checkmark, 2004), 381.

8 Umberto Eco, *Six Walks in the Fictional Woods* (Cambridge, MA: Harvard University Press, 1995), 52. For his adaptation of the novel, see Eco, *The Story of the Betrothed*, trans. Stephen Sartarelli, ill. Marcoi Lorenzetti (London: Pushkin Children's Books, 2017).

respect to the time in which they are set that they would have seemed probable even to people of that time, had the novel been written for them."[9] To write with verisimilitude is to write what Plato called "likely stories." Manzoni envisioned his own function as writer as a balance between the imaginative and the factual, the poet and the historian. The historical novelist writes what never happened in keeping with what *could* have happened and what historical patterns suggest was the most probable turn of events, given the particular circumstances invented by the author. In describing the 1630 plague and its consequences, Manzoni (as both poet and historian) must begin with concrete facts and statistics and deduce their effect on imagined characters of certain types. However, a perfect synthesis of the dual roles of the historical novelist is never possible: "A great poet and a great historian may be found in the same man without creating confusion, but not in the same work."[10]

The general plot of *The Betrothed* is simple and strikes us as quaintly romantic today. The drama begins in 1628, with Milan under the despotic rule of Spain. Renzo Tramaglino and Lucia Mondella are a young, betrothed peasant couple living in Lombardy. The day before their nuptials, the priest who is to officiate, Don Abbondio, is approached by two bravos and told, "There's not going to be any marriage, not tomorrow nor any other day" (8).[11] The local Spanish baron, Don Rodrigo, has forbidden this marriage to take place. Don Rodrigo is himself taken with Lucia, and has made a wager with his cousin, Count Attilio, that he shall possess her by the feast of St. Martin. When Don Rodrigo eventually sends armed men to seize Lucia, she and Renzo manage to evade capture and flee from home with the aid of Fra Cristoforo, a Capuchin with "the reputation of a saint" (123). Lucia is placed in a convent in Monza, while Renzo is relocated to Milan, stricken at the time by famine.

From this beginning, the separated pair has a series of adventures and misadventures before they are finally reunited. Don Rodrigo and Count Attilio continue their scheming; Renzo is arrested but manages to escape; Lucia is abducted by a notorious bandit, the "Unnamed," as part of Rodrigo's plan, but he has a sudden change of heart, publicly renounces villainy, and sees her safely home. While she is being held by the "Unnamed," Lucia makes an unfortunate vow that further complicates the

9 Alessandro Manzoni, *On the Historical Novel*, trans. Sandra Bermann (Lincoln, NE: University of Nebraska Press, 1984), 125.

10 Ibid., 126.

11 All parenthetical citations in this section refer to Alessandro Manzoni, *The Betrothed*, trans. Archibald Colquhoun (New York: E. P. Dutton & Co., 1961).

plight of the young lovers. In despair, she swears to the Virgin Mary, "Rescue me from this danger, take me back safely to my mother, oh, Mother of the Lord! and I make a vow to you to remain a virgin; I renounce my poor Renzo for ever, in order to be henceforth yours and yours alone" (322).

Throughout all of these scenes, there is the airy lightness of the adventure novels of Dumas or Henry Fielding. The stakes are high for the two main characters, but one knows that one is not reading a Greek tragedy; the couple must be united again after all these mishaps. Suddenly, the direction of the narrative is violently cut through by the outbreak of the Great Plague in 1630, and all values are reorganized as the novel takes on a funereal tone. For two chapters, our heroes are not once mentioned, as Manzoni (in keeping with his own principles) abandons poetry in order to become a historian. The lesson for us to draw today from the plague scenes in *The Betrothed* is that *crises disrupt the course of life, and present an opportunity for forgiveness and the reorganization of passions*.

Chapters 31 through 33 of *The Betrothed* contain Manzoni's description of the plague. His interest in the 1630 pandemic continued well past the initial composition of *The Betrothed*. In 1842, Manzoni included a historical essay, *The History of the Infamous Column* (*La storia della colonna infame*), as an appendix to a revised edition of *The Betrothed*. The *Infamous Column* deals with a particular event mentioned briefly in *The Betrothed*, namely the affair of certain "anointers" of Milan, suspected of applying ointment to the houses of Milan to spread the plague (501–4). Manzoni's primary source for information about the plague was *La peste di Milano del 1630*, a first-hand account written by Giuseppe Ripamonti, professor of rhetoric and "the official chronicler of the history of Milan."[12] However, this was not his only source, and he admits a desire to correct a failure of all historians and compose the first "clear and connected" account of the plague (470). He writes, "We have only tried to bring out and to verify the most general and important facts, to arrange them in the real order in which they happened, so far as reason and their nature will allow, to observe their influence on each other, and to give for the present, and until someone else does it better, a succinct, but honest and continuous, account of the disaster" (471).

In Manzoni's narrative, he relates how the plague was brought to Milan by an Italian soldier in the service of Spain. The Milanese Tribunal of Health was quick to respond, quarantining the man and his family and

12 Giorgio A. Pinton, *The Conspiracy of the Prince of Macchia & G. B. Vico* (New York: Rodopi, 2013), 187.

having his household goods burned. However, they could not keep his attending nurses from infection, and the severe measures adopted by the Tribunal kept the sick from reporting their symptoms in a timely manner. There was also resistance amongst public health officials against calling the plague by name or announcing an epidemic, which hindered preventative measures. This suppression of evidence of epidemics is common to many historical outbreaks, the present one included. As Robert Fletcher observes, "To declare that the plague had appeared in Milan was to drive the people off, and to frighten trade away."[13] Herd blindness set in amongst an incredulous population, who had not faced a serious plague epidemic for nearly two generations. However, the Milanese could not be kept ignorant of the outbreak forever, and "toward the end of the month of March the cases of illness, of death with strange spasms, palpitations, coma, delirium, and those fatal symptoms of livid spots and tumours, began to grow frequent" (479). Both magistrates and the public at large were compelled to overcome their obstinacy and admit the presence of a very real medical crisis. The Tribunal eventually took drastic measures to alert the public, having the corpses of a family that had all perished of plague drawn naked through a large gathering, "so that the crowds could see the obvious marks of pestilence on them" (485–86).

From this beginning, Manzoni descends into the wretched situation in Milan as the plague flourished. The *lazzaretto*, an enormous hospital that was set up to accommodate two thousand patients, soon had a population of sixteen thousand. The death rate in the city alone soon exceeded five hundred a day, and reached as high as twelve or fifteen hundred a day. The exact statistics are varied, but Manzoni cites solid research claiming "the number of deaths on the civic registers came to one hundred and forty thousand, apart from those that could not be counted" (494). When the large public grave that was dug near the hospital was filled with corpses, bodies began to be left rotting on the streets. Food was often scarce, exacerbated by the famine from which Milan had only just recovered. Villainy increased, as it always does in crises: "Rogues whom the plague spared and did not frighten found new chances of activity, together with new certainty of impunity, in the common confusion following the relaxation of every public authority; in fact the very exercise of public authority came to be in the hands of the worst among them" (497). As crime grew, so did panic. Panic, we have seen, is the abandonment of rationality as the

13 Robert Fletcher, *A Tragedy of the Great Plague of Milan in 1630* (Baltimore: The Lord Baltimore Press, 1898), 14.

primary instrument of thought and action. A public that responds with panic to a crisis is prone to compound its errors in judgment.

When we are finally reintroduced to our heroes, we find them suffering just as much as the rest of northern Italy. Count Attilio, we are told in passing, has died, "carried off by the plague two days before" (505). After delighting the mourners with a comic funeral oration, Don Rodrigo, the book's primary antagonist, begins to feel uneasy: "a heaviness, a weakness of the legs, a difficulty in breathing, a burning feeling inside him," his face distorted and inflamed (505). He awakens from a restless sleep to a throbbing pain in his side, and discovers the token of certain death, "a hideous tumour of livid purple hue" (507). Renzo and Lucia's implacable adversary, whose machinations have terrorized their hopes for happiness, is disarmed by the sudden fell stroke of pestilence. The novel's main source of dramatic tension is disrupted and resolved at once. The troubles of the heroes are not resolved by any actions they take on their own behalf, as one would expect in a romance.[14] The malicious genius of the novel ingloriously falls victim to the plague, which does not discriminate heroes from villains.

At the same time, Renzo is likewise stricken by the pandemic. "Renzo caught the plague, too, and cured himself—that is, he did nothing. He was at death's door from it, but his strong constitution defeated the disease; in a few days he was out of danger" (512). The 1630 plague was wildly contagious, but contagion was fatal in only around half of all cases. In itself, this is a gloomy survival rate, but by comparison it was substantially less fatal than the Black Death three centuries earlier. Renzo, young and robust, managed to survive, whereas his older, more hedonistic and sedentary adversaries did not. As a survivor, he entered a "privileged class among the rest of the population," the small class able to move about freely with the confidence of inoculation (514). After much journeying through the countryside in search of Lucia, and beholding the devastation wrought in his native village by the plague, Renzo receives word that she too has fallen ill and is one of the tens of thousands of patients at the over-filled *lazzaretto* in Milan. There he finds the good Fra Cristoforo tending to the stricken, having felt it his duty "to give his life for his fellow-creatures" (548). Cristoforo himself soon succumbs without fanfare, as anonymous

14 Benedetto Croce has noted differences in type between the historical romanticism of Scott and the "historical fiction of Manzoni, which is free from such sentiment and whose historical element has a moral foundation." *History, Its Theory and Practice*, trans. Douglas Ainslie (New York: Harcourt, Brace and Co., 1921), 265.

in death as Don Rodrigo. Renzo is finally reunited with a recovering Lucia, whose vow to remain celibate is absolved by Fra Cristoforo, and the two are wed at last by Don Abbondio, their nuptials having been delayed by two years.

One can imagine the pair of convalescents, ashen and weak, their peasant vitality greatly diminished by their deathly sickness, their faces no longer beaming with either beauty or innocence. They slowly discover together which friends and family members remain living and which have perished. They are married in the end, giving the novel a happy ending and placing it in the traditional category of comedy. However, these are not the same characters that are betrothed when the novel begins, and their happiness is undermined by the loss of everything but each other. They do not enter as one into a world they know, but into a world that they must now build anew. Their final reflections carry a note of Greek tragedy: "That troubles often come to those who bring them on themselves, but that not even the most cautious and innocent behavior can ward them off; and that when they come—whether by our own fault or not—confidence in God can lighten them and turn them to our own improvement" (604). The modern tragic hero brings suffering upon himself. Greek tragedies are woven into the fabric of the cosmos, and are inescapable, however virtuously and correctly one behaves. Plague has the force of Greek tragedy, and though Renzo and Lucia survive, the style of their characters must transform and evolve. They must reorder their foundational ideas and values.

We see this illustrated in a poignant scene at the *lazzaretto*, where Renzo is brought face to face with the dying Don Rodrigo, his enemy and tormenter. Leading up to this encounter, Renzo vents his rage in violent language: "If the fellow's still alive, I'll find him. … The time's come when men meet each other face to face; and … I'll do my own justice, I will!" (552). Fra Cristoforo remonstrates with Renzo for his resentment, cautioning that his temper is hateful to God. "You can hate, and be lost; you can, with that feeling in you, alienate every blessing from yourself. For, however things go with you, however much you prosper, you can be sure that it will all turn into a penance until you have forgiven him" (554). Renzo reflects on this lecture, and is then brought before Don Rodrigo. Rodrigo's eyes are sightless, his face "pale and covered with black blotches, his lips black and swollen," and his body convulses with occasional spasms, the only sign of life the wretched body evinces. Renzo renounces his rage with a silent gesture, bowing his face over Rodrigo and praying for the man (555). Love replaces wrath, and Renzo's heart is divided between thoughts of Rodrigo and Lucia (557).

This is not inconstancy of character. The Stoics viewed constancy as one of the foremost virtues. The Renaissance neo-Stoic Justus Lipsius argued that constancy is the proper attitude in the face of disasters like plague, which occur in all ages. He defines constancy as the "right and immovable strength of mind, neither lifted up nor pressed down with external or casual accidents." However, he excludes from this definition obstinacy, "which is a certain hardness of a stubborn mind, proceeding from pride or vainglory."[15] When he offers as consolation for suffering his observations on pandemics—"Tell me, how many thousands have died of the pestilence in all the Low Countries within these five or six years? I think fifty or at the most one hundred thousand. But one plague in Judea in the time of king David swept away seventy thousand in less space than one whole day"[16]—he is not advocating for hard-heartedness. The constant mind is that which does not abandon reason, and is guided in its behavior by sound judgment rather than passion. The character that does not reorganize its values and emotions in light of a disaster is not constant, but proud and stubborn.

Pandemics are destabilizing catastrophes for the individuals who survive their ravages. As has been shown, they are the sort of crisis that instigates wholesale revaluation of one's integral character. New modes of apprehending the world arise, and new organizations of the passions are necessary for adaptation. The survivor must *evolve*. If we are to draw an applicable lesson from Manzoni's brilliant character study, it is that it behooves us to subject our foundational attitudes to new scrutiny. Is the set of things that mattered to us yesterday still meaningful today? or has the abrupt disruption of all norms created novel circumstances under which it becomes prudent to behave differently? Every change in circumstances requires alterations in how we understand the good life and how we act to achieve it. Drastic changes of the one call for equally drastic revisions of the other. We are compelled to reorganize our basic impulses and passions. In the words of José Ortega y Gasset, "I am myself plus my circumstance, and if I do not save it, I cannot save myself."[17]

For all of us, there are human beings that we dislike, and some of us may harbor anger and wrath and treasure a thirst for vengeance. These

15 Justus Lipsius, *On Constancy*, trans. Sir John Stradling, ed. John Sellars (Exeter: Bristol Phoenix Press, 2006), 37.

16 Ibid., 120.

17 José Ortega y Gasset, *Meditations on Quixote*, trans. Evelyn Rugg and Diego Marín (Urbana, IL: University of Illinois Press, 2000), 45.

feelings have their bases in concrete events. They are responses one deems appropriate, taking into consideration a vast complex of personal and social factors. One takes offense at a hostile word. In the background of this response are fixed ideas about norms of social decorum; about one's relationship to the speaker or the two parties' respective roles within greater organizations; about what degree of insult one's dignity is able to tolerate without diminution; and so on. Crisis upsets these ideas. The broken body of Rodrigo—like the broken body of Kuragin in Tolstoy's *War and Peace*—reminds us that the enemies we elevate in our minds to the status of monsters are in fact merely men and women. Have you been offended by a scoundrel? Very well. Does not this pandemic affect you both, indiscriminately, without regard to right and wrong? If you are able to evolve and adapt to the new situation of the world, do these offenses still carry the same meaning, or is your outrage now a product of inertia? Manzoni counsels us to forgive.

If our anger derives from a feeling of pain, it has no basis when then pain diminishes or is effaced by other worries. When the crisis situation abates and social institutions settle into new patterns of regularity, our personal projects must likewise change to meet these new contingencies. Reason demands that we adapt and evolve. Constancy itself demands malleability. It is irrational for an evolving mind to fixate on emotions that have lost their foundations. The retention of animosities that are groundless within one's new social paradigm is folly, just as the retention of friendships without ground is folly. To remain fixated on old slights is, as Lipsius says, "pride and vainglory." It impedes the evolution of one's character and undermines one's ability to form new passions applicable to a restructured world. To follow the lesson of Manzoni is to take the occasion of crisis to reassess one's emotions, and to abandon the dead matter of ancient indignation.

CHAPTER VII

Thomas Mann

Death in Venice

Restrain the Passionate Life

Friedrich Nietzsche's philological essay *The Birth of Tragedy*, written in 1872, interpreted dramatic art in an unprecedented manner. Nietzsche was a scholar of language and antiquities, and he is at his best as a commentator on Greek thought. Nietzsche spent his lifetime confronting what he saw as the rising specter of nihilism that threatened to consume Europe. In Athenian tragedy, he found a form of art that overcomes the pessimism born of the sense of meaninglessness. His great discovery was what he termed the "Dionysian" element of Greek thought. He argues that Athenian tragedy is the result of a dialectical meeting of the Dionysian and Apollonian worldviews. To rediscover the spirit of Greek tragedy is the salvation of the human spirit in a nihilistic age: "Yes, my friends, believe with me in Dionysian life and the rebirth of tragedy. The age of the Socratic man is over. ... Only dare to be tragic men; for you are to be redeemed."[1]

In Nietzsche's theory, the Apollonian and Dionysian viewpoints are diametrically opposed. Apollo is the god of the sun, rational thought, and wisdom; he is the embodiment of logic and prudence. Dionysus is the youngest of the divinities, the half-caste stranger from the east, who represents wine and song, and whose cult emphasizes sensuality and passion over reason, frenzy over order. Dionysus brings to the stolid, rational Greeks the lightness of the vine. As the seer Teiresias says in Euripides, Dionysus is one of two great blessings to humankind. First is Demeter, the source of grain,

> But after her came the son of Semele [Dionysus],
> who matched her present by inventing liquid wine
> as his gift to man. For filled with that good gift,
> suffering mankind forgets its grief.[2]

Nietzsche writes that Apollo is the symbol of "measured restraint, that

1 Friedrich Nietzsche, *The Birth of Tragedy and The Case of Wagner*, trans. Walter Kaufmann (New York: Vintage, 1967), 124.

2 Euripides, *The Bacchae*, trans. William Arrowsmith, in *Euripides V*, ed. David Grene and Richmond Lattimore (Chicago: University of Chicago Press, 1968), lines 277–80.

freedom from the wilder emotions, that calm of the sculptor god. His eye must be 'sunlike,' as befits his origin; even when it is angry and distempered it is still hallowed by beautiful illusion." Dionysus, on the other hand, brings the collapse of the boundaries between appearance and reality. "Either under the influence of narcotic draught … or with the potent coming of spring that penetrates all nature with joy, these Dionysian emotions awake, and as they grow in intensity everything subjective vanishes into complete self-forgetfulness." Rationalism frowns upon what it perceives as the madness of the Bacchae, and yet "such poor wretches have no idea how corpselike and ghostly their so-called 'healthy-mindedness' looks when the glowing life of the Dionysian roars past them."[3] The Apollonian spirit builds a clearly demarcated world in which all things have their distinct place, oneself included. The Dionysian spirit returns all things to primordial unity.

For Nietzsche, Greek tragedy is the result of the fusion of these two spirits. The idealized, plastic art of the Apollonian viewpoint meets with the unfettered Dionysian viewpoint of festival and song on the Athenian stage. The Dionysian element is the tragic chorus of satyrs, in which "the Greek man of culture felt himself nullified." The satyrs exist is a world of myth. The immediate effect of the Dionysian chorus is that "the state and society and, quite generally, the gulfs between man and man give way to an overwhelming feeling of unity leading back to the very heart of nature." However, the choral parts are more of a guiding thread than the heart of the tragedy. Nietzsche refers to them as "the womb that gave birth to the whole of the so-called dialogue, that is, the entire world of the stage, the real drama."[4] The dialogue of the actors on stage, with its concrete symbolic meaning, is the Apollonian element. Dionysian insight, which is attuned to "primal being," is the source of the drama, but is abstract and raw. Apollonian intellectualism gives form to this insight through the self-controlled dialogue of the staged drama. Because Greek tragedy is able to balance the demands of the two primal instincts of humankind, it embraces the whole of the human condition. Nietzsche holds that authentic tragedy died with Sophocles, and that later artists were unable to strike the same balance between intellect and emotion. In 1872 he was optimistic that Richard Wagner might personify a rebirth of tragedy, but in later years he was thoroughly disillusioned about this prospect.

Thomas Mann (1875–1955) was the most important German author

3 Nietzsche, *Birth of Tragedy*, 35–37.
4 Ibid., 59; 65.

of the twentieth century. He was awarded the Nobel Prize for Literature in 1929 and the Goethe Prize in 1949. Though he lived through two world wars and the slow barbarization of the Germanic spirit, Mann remained the world's foremost voice of German culture throughout his life. His work was greatly informed by the thought of the great artists and philosophers of Germany's past, in particular Nietzsche and Johann Wolfgang von Goethe. Nietzsche was a model for the humanist Lodovico Settembrini in *The Magic Mountain*, and his thought is reflected in the character and attitudes of Adrian Leverkühn, protagonist of *Doctor Faustus*. *Doctor Faustus* is also a modern retelling of the Faust legend popularized in Germany by Goethe, and Goethe is a model for Gustave von Aschenbach, protagonist of *Death in Venice*. Mann, like Nietzsche, tended to think in terms of opposed dualisms (art versus life; the individual versus society). His literary output was in part shaped by the dualism of Goethe and Nietzsche, the former representing to Mann the cosmopolitan aesthete, the latter the reclusive realist; the former the poet as intellectual, the latter the intellectual as poet.

Mann's most widely read work today is his 1912 novella *Death in Venice* (*Der Tod in Venedig*). This short book narrates the final days of a respected middle-aged German writer named Gustave von Aschenbach. Suffering from writer's block, Aschenbach decides on a change of scenery and takes a vacation in Venice. At his hotel, he notices a boy of around fourteen and is taken by "the lad's perfect beauty," in keeping with "the noblest moment in Greek sculpture" (25).[5] On the beach, Aschenbach again beholds the boy with great interest, and overhears his name, Tadzio. As Aschenbach's health begins to decline, he resolves to leave Venice, but he cannot bring himself to do so. Weeks pass, and his obsession with Tadzio grows. One evening, Tadzio smiles at Aschenbach, and the event is overwhelming. The old author flees into the abandoned garden and, in a stupor far beneath his dignity, "whispered the hackneyed phrase of love and longing—impossible in these circumstances, absurd, abject, ridiculous enough, yet sacred too, and not unworthy of honour even here: 'I love you!'" (51).

While Aschenbach's homoerotic attraction to Tadzio develops into an unhealthy fixation, it becomes increasingly evident that a public health crisis is imminent in Venice. German newspapers report an unnamed

5 All parenthetical references in this section refer to Thomas Mann, *Death in Venice*, in *Death in Venice and Seven Other Stories*, trans. H. T. Lowe-Porter (New York: Vintage, 1989), 45.

pestilence striking Venice and suggest contradictory death totals, though Venetian authorities deny any such crisis. The streets of Venice are disinfected, but the official position is that it is merely a precaution against the sirocco, the hot winds: "A plague? What sort of plague? Is the sirocco a plague?" (60). Aschenbach finally discovers that the city is in the midst of a cholera outbreak. He considers warning Tadzio's family so that they can escape in time, but keeps silent because cannot bear the thought of the boy's leaving. Aschenbach stalks Tadzio's movements, his behavior becoming increasingly erratic and ridiculous, although he never speaks a word to the boy or makes his feelings known. Finally, he learns one day that Tadzio and his family are leaving to return home. Heartbroken, he goes down to the beach, where he sees Tadzio one final time, his gaze lingering on the boy's breast, and there Aschenbach dies, a victim of the cholera he failed to take precautions against.

Death in Venice explores in concrete narrative the Nietzschean idea of the conflict between Apollonian and Dionysian impulses. When the story begins, Aschenbach is the consummate Apollonian intellectual. He is introduced as an austere and conscientious man in his mid-fifties, leading a life governed by a severe "pattern of self-discipline he had followed from his youth up" (6). However, undergoing what we might now call a mid-life crisis, he finds himself grappling with an unfamiliar "contagion" of the spirit: "This yearning for new and distant scenes, this craving for freedom, release, forgetfulness—they were, he admitted to himself, an impulse towards flight, flight from the spot which was the daily theatre of a rigid, cold, and passionate service." Aschenbach is devoted to his labor and duty, "the enervating daily struggle between a proud, tenacious, well-tried will and this growing fatigue, which no one must suspect." However, he finds it impossible to resist or to "suppress summarily a need that so unequivocally asserted itself," the call of the Dionysian (6–7). He therefore leaves his home and his rigidly organized life in Munich for Venice, a city of *gondole*, romance, and danger, the setting of the eternal struggle between Othello and Iago.

As Aschenbach's obsession with Tadzio develops, he is thrown off-balance and progressively sacrifices logical thought to the demands of his emergent passions. In his sober moments of self-control, Aschenbach recognizes his folly and seriously entertains "the thought of returning home, returning to reason, self-mastery, an ordered existence, to the old life and effort." However, he quickly rejects this impulse in favor of the passionate life, and "the bare thought made him wince with a revulsion that was like physical nausea" (65). The novella is steeped in allusions to Greek philosophy and mythology, which form a symbolic framework for the story and cast Aschenbach as an initiate in the bacchic mysteries. Reflecting on the longing that arises in his heart, Aschenbach muses, "Should we not perish and be consumed by love, as Semele aforetime was by Zeus?" (45). Semele is the human mother of Dionysus, who was consumed in flame when she demanded to behold the true form of her lover Zeus. Even Aschenbach's dreams become Dionysian in character. Mann describes dreams of frenzied orgies amidst sweet flute music, in which "he heard a voice, naming, though darkly, that which was to come: 'The stranger god!' … From the wooded heights, from among the tree-trunks and crumbling moss-covered rocks, a troop came tumbling and raging down, a whirling rout of men and animals, and overflowed the hillside with flames and human forms, with clamour and the reeling dance" (65–66). "The stranger God" is Dionysus himself—the stranger from the east—and the raucous troop is the Bacchae, his votaries. Aschenbach slowly sacrifices his dignified self-control to the frenzied, passionate life of the Dionysian cult.

In his correspondence, Mann writes to Carl Maria Weber about the central dualism of *Death in Venice*. He says, "It is inherent in the difference between the Dionysian spirit of lyricism, whose outpouring is irresponsible and individualistic, and the Apollonian, objectively controlled, morally and socially responsible epic. What I was after was an equilibrium of sensuality and morality. … But that the novella is at its core of a hymnic type, indeed of hymnic origin, cannot have escaped you." Mann confesses that his own biases compelled him to see the case in "a pathological light," and that like the characters in the story he himself is limited by an "altogether non-'Greek' but rather Protestant, Puritan ('bourgeois') basic state of mind … in other words, our fundamentally mistrustful, fundamentally pessimistic relationship to passion in general."[6] Aschenbach is the model puritan, the model bourgeoisie, who finds himself shattered upon the rocks of emerging passion.

The Venetian outbreak of cholera in the background of the story mirrors the personal crisis of Aschenbach. The disintegration and frenzy of his own spirit is reflected broadly in the medical crisis of the romantic city. As the story progresses, the danger posed by this epidemic becomes more and more evident. The official explanation is that there is nothing to fear,

6 Thomas Mann, Letter to Carl Maria Weber (4 July 1920), in *Letters of Thomas Mann, 1889–1955*, trans. Richard and Clara Winston (Los Angeles: University of California Press, 1975), 93–94.

"a mere formality. Quite regular in view of the unhealthy climatic conditions." However, Aschenbach learns from a clerk at an English travel bureau that there is more to the outbreak than this. A pernicious strand of cholera has devastated Asia for some time, originating in the Ganges region, moving through China with great violence, and bringing "terror to Astrakhan, terror to Moscow." Europe "trembled" in dread of infection as the disease began to appear in port cities along the Mediterranean. It soon broke out in several southern Italian cities, though northern Italy was for a time spared. However, "In May the horrible vibrions were found on the same day in two bodies: the emaciated, blackened corpses of a bargee and a woman who kept a green-grocer's shop. Both cases were hushed up. But in a week there were ten more—twenty, thirty in different quarters of the town." Authorities continued to deny the existence of a crisis, but "by that time the food supplies—milk, meat, or vegetables—had probably been contaminated, for death unseen and unacknowledged was devouring and laying waste in the narrow streets, while a brooding, unseasonable heat warmed the waters of the canals and encouraged the spread of the pestilence" (62–63).

Venice did in fact suffer an outbreak of cholera in 1911, which was part of a larger, global pandemic, though Mann does not write his novella as a true historical account, and he gives no more precise date for the events of the book than "19—." Venetian officials carefully suppressed the truth about the severity of the outbreak for as long as they were able. Official releases from Venice say that 116 people died of cholera in 1911. However, a report of the Provincial Officer of Health suggests that the true figures were concealed by authorities. He reports that in a five month period, "the province had suffered 778 reported cases of cholera, of which 605 had been bacteriologically confirmed, and 262 deaths—more than double the 'official' total."[7] In *Death in Venice*, the cholera outbreak is much more fatal than this. Mann writes, "Recoveries were rare. Eighty out of every hundred died, and horribly, for the onslaught was of the extremest violence, and not infrequently of the 'dry' type, the most malignant form of the contagion. In this form the victim's body loses power to expel the water secreted by the blood-vessels, it shrivels up, he passes with hoarse cries from convulsion to convulsion, his blood grows thick like pitch, and he suffocates in a few hours." In more fortunate cases, "the disease, after a slight *malaise*, takes the form of a profound unconsciousness, from

7 Frank M. Snowden, *Naples in the Time of Cholera, 1884–1911* (New York: Cambridge University Press, 2002), 327.

which the sufferer seldom or never rouses" (63). As the population comes more and more to recognize the existence of this outbreak, there is a marked rise in indecency and crime. "Theft and assault were said to be frequent, even murder" (64).

Because of his erotic longing and the renunciation of Apollonian prudence, Aschenbach fails to take action and leave the stricken city while possible, or shelter himself in safety. He unnecessarily becomes a victim of the epidemic, dying alone and unfulfilled like the hollow men of T. S. Eliot: "This is the way the world ends / Not with a bang but a whimper."[8] He is taken in the midst of his reveries, by the form of the disease that brings unconsciousness without recovery. Mann writes his inglorious end with the minimal fanfare it deserves: "Some minutes passed before anyone hastened to the aid of the elderly man sitting there collapsed in his chair. They bore him to his room. And before nightfall a shocked and respectful world received the news of his decease" (73).

Death in Venice portrays Aschenbach not as a model for prudent behavior, but as a cautionary tale. Mann characterized the theme of the novella as the danger of the Dionysian impulses. He writes, "Passion as confusion and as a stripping of dignity was really the subject of my tale—what I originally wanted to deal with was not anything homoerotic at all. It was the story—seen grotesquely—of the aged Goethe and that little girl in Marienbad whom he was absolutely determined to marry, with the acquiescence of her social-climbing procuress of a mother and despite the outraged horror of his own family, with the girl not wanting it at all—this story with all its terribly comic, shameful, awesomely ridiculous situations, the embarrassing, touching, and grandiose story."[9] Passion is portrayed at its most reckless and embarrassing in this story, and connected with the loss of dignity. The Dionysian reveler is without restraint and without self-awareness. In the throes of the revel, the individual personality is nullified. The bacchant becomes capable of anything, however inhuman. In Euripides, the princess Agave, under the sway of Dionysus, tears her son Pentheus limb from limb, mistaking him for a mountain lion, and holds his head up proudly, announcing, "Happy was the hunting."[10] Aschenbach's descent is made more pathetic by his occasional moments of clarity, in which he recognizes himself as Agave. In his dreams, "It was he … who bit and tore and swallowed smoking gobbets of flesh—while

8 T. S. Eliot, "The Hollow Men," in *Complete Poems*, 59.
9 Mann, Letter to Weber, 94–95.
10 Euripides, *Bacchae*, line 1171.

on the trampled moss there now began the rites in honour of the god, an orgy of promiscuous embraces—and in his very soul he tasted the bestial degradation of his fall" (67).

Mann's counsel for pandemics is negative: *Do not allow the Dionysian impulses to gain the upper hand.* This could be phrased differently as *restrain the passionate element of life.* We have seen repeatedly in our other authors that plague situations have a tendency to loosen the inhibitions of some individuals. Pandemics often bring about a fatalistic mentality that manifests itself in an increase in crime and a decrease in modesty. Reason loses its hegemony as its promise of stability is undermined by concrete events. Under normal conditions, it is clear that rational self-control is the best strategy for long-term wellbeing. During a crisis, however, this reason for embracing rationalism evaporates. As Scripture says, "Let us eat and drink, for tomorrow we die."[11] This is fine advice for the prisoner awaiting execution, but it is by no means so certain that any one in particular will be the victim of a pandemic. Living well during an outbreak requires the rejection of this pessimistic outlook. Right action always necessitates self-discipline and the guidance of reason. To relinquish this is to relinquish one's basic dignity and to exchange order for confusion.

The romance of Goethe that Mann mentions, and which he used as inspiration for his Aschenbach character, was not the finest moment in the life of that lion of German culture. At the age of seventy-two, Goethe became enamored with the seventeen-year-old Baroness Ulrike von Levetzow. When she rejected his proposal of marriage, he addressed a trilogy of poems to her in which he admits his befuddled state of mind:

> And 'twas through *her!*—an inward sorrow lay
> On soul and body, heavily oppressed;
> To mournful phantoms was my sight a prey,
> In the drear void of a sad tortured breast.

Goethe's elegy ends with his lament that the gods, who once showed him favor, "urged me to those lips, with rapture crowned, / Deserted me, and hurled me to the ground."[12] The undignified infatuation of the aged poet—the man who composed *The Sorrows of Young Werther* and *Faust*, and gave shape and direction to German national character in the nineteenth century—is hauntingly pathetic.

---

11 Isa. 22:13.

12 Johann Wolfgang von Goethe, "[Marienbad] Elegy," in *The Poems of Goethe*, trans. E. A. Browning et al (New York: Thomas Y. Crowell & Co., 1882), 205; 206.

Early in *Death in Venice*, while crossing to Italy by ship, Aschenbach sees an old man amidst a group of virile youths, and feels ashamed for this fop, thinking him "a truly repulsive sight" (19). The old man debases himself with the façade of youth, dressing himself up in "a dandified buff suit, a rakish panama with a coloured scarf, and a red cravat." Aschenbach shudders and muses, "Could they not see he was old, that he had no right to wear the clothes they wore or pretend to be one of them?" (17). However, at his most ridiculous, Aschenbach himself becomes this old fool. He finds himself desperately trying to recover his youthfulness and faded beauty, in order to attract the pubescent Tadzio. He brightens and ornaments his dress and begins to pay frequent visits to the hotel barber. He has his hair died, his lips tinted, and his face cosmetically made up in powder and rouge. This is the very image of foppery, this genteel old man dandified and painted, fooling only himself with the mask of vitality. This is Goethe in his dotage, the lion in winter, being made a fool while pining in unrequited love for a child. This is Pentheus in *The Bacchae*, who so proudly defies the indecency of the Bacchic cult for a time but in the end, longing to behold the secrets of Dionysius, allows himself to me made up as a woman, in female dress and fine furs, his hair done up in long curls by Dionysius himself.[13] All three, from admirable men, are transformed into laughingstocks when the Dionysian impulses get the better of the Apollonian.

Aschenbach is not, however, the enormous personality that Goethe was. He is much more an image of Mann himself. Harold Bloom writes, "The painstaking artist Mann is darkly conscious that he lacks the Goethean spontaneity, the sublime excess of a charismatic personality. One can conceive Goethe as a Shakespearean character, but not Thomas Mann."[14] Goethe's was an enormous personality, and Goethe's Faust is a character on par with Don Quixote, an individual who personifies everything wonderful and terrible in the human spirit. Faust is a man who bargains with devils and sleeps with Helen of Troy. Mann's characters are all essentially ordinary. This power of creating ordinary heroes is one of Mann's strengths as a writer. Hans Castorp is the everyman, and we relate to *The Magic Mountain* because we are all Hans Castorp and the mountain is everywhere. Thomas Buddenbrook, the protagonist for much of *Buddenbrooks*, collapses and dies in the street after a botched dental

---

13 Euripides, *Bacchae*, lines 828–38.

14 Harold Bloom, *Genius: A Mosaic of One Hundred Exemplary Creative Minds* (New York: Warner Books, 2002), 186.

procedure—a far cry from the storm and stress death of Goethe's young Werther. Aschenbach, too, is ordinary, a respectable man who lives an upright life but succumbs to passion and pays the cost with his life.

This ordinariness makes the tragedy of Gustave von Aschenbach more relevant to our own lives than the sublime characters of Goethe. From Aschenbach, the reader learns the prudent lesson of avoiding excess and maintaining spiritual equilibrium. Most of us are not made to strive for the passionless life of the anchorite. Passion gives life its content and its pulse. However, as is the case on the Athenian stage, it is the self-controlled Apollonian intellect that must give form to passion. If a fusion is required for art to reach its highest perfection, a similar fusion is required for human life to reach its highest artistry. In Munich, Aschenbach is too much the Apollonian, going through life "corpselike," to use Nietzsche's phrase. In Venice, he becomes too much the Dionysian, and the cost is the self-discipline that makes him respected in the world. The release of long-repressed energies cripples the organism's normal functioning. Aschenbach even valorizes his own wretchedness, telling himself, "Many heroes of olden time had willingly borne his yoke, not counting any humiliation such if it happened by [Eros'] decree; vows, protestations, self-abasements, these were no source of shame to the lover" (57).

Prudent action in times of pandemics need not be passionless. Strozzi and Machiavelli show us that it remains possible even amidst the plague to discover erotic passion, and that this vital aspect of the inner life should not be denied. To give the passions free reign, however, is to be guided not by thought, but by the chthonic energies of the unconscious. This makes us subordinate what is best to what is desired. Platonic *eros* is sympathy between minds. The true lover leaves the vicinity of the plague and ensures that his beloved safely escapes also, even should they never meet again. It is only a ridiculous fool who risks infection in himself and the beloved so that he may behold the latter's shirtless torso from afar once or twice more. The good life includes much passion, but not at in place of sound judgment.

The most enduring philosophical image of the relationship between intellect and passion is the chariot analogy in Plato's *Phaedrus*. The *Phaedrus* is an erotic dialogue about the nature of love, throughout which runs a flirtation between Socrates and his young interlocutor Phaedrus. In his inner monologue, Aschenbach refers to Tadzio as Phaedrus several times, referencing the themes of the dialogue: "For beauty, my Phædrus, beauty alone, is lovely and visible at once. For, mark you, it is the sole aspect of the spiritual which we can perceive through our senses. … So beauty, then, is the beauty-lover's way to the spirit—but only the way, only the means, my little Phædrus" (44–45).

In the *Phaedrus*, Socrates says, "Let us then liken the soul to the natural union of a team of winged horses and their charioteer. … To begin with, our driver is in charge of a pair of horses; second, one of his horses is beautiful and good and from stock of the same sort, while the other is the opposite and has the opposite sort of bloodline. This means that chariot-driving in our case is inevitably a painfully difficult business."[15] The charioteer is the individual's intellect or reason, which must guide the team in the right direction. The good horse is the spirited part of the soul, which is attracted by proper objects of desire. The other, the "dark horse," is the irrational, appetitive part of the soul, governed only by hedonistic desire. In Freudian psychoanalysis, these three divisions of the soul are termed Superego, Ego, and Id, respectively. The wings of the horses are *Eros*, which has the power to lift the soul. These wings are nourished by beauty, goodness, and wisdom, but baseness and ugliness make the wings shrink and disappear. Socrates says, "The heaviness of the bad horse drags its charioteer toward the earth and weighs him down if he has failed to train it well, and this causes the most extreme toil and struggle that a soul will face."[16] The aim of the charioteer is to ascend beyond the heavens to a place where one can apprehend reality with the mind. Here, the soul "is delighted at last to be seeing what is real and watching what is true. … On the way around it has a view of Justice as it is; it has a view of Self-control; it has a view of Knowledge. … And when the soul has seen all the things that are as they are and feasted on them, it sinks back inside heaven and goes home."[17]

For the chariot to succeed in this ascent, the proper order must be maintained between horses and charioteer. The good horse is a "lover of honor with modesty and self-control; companion to true glory, he needs no whip, and is guided by verbal commands alone. The other horse is a crooked great jumble of limbs … companion to wild boasts and indecency, he is shaggy around the ears—deaf as a post—and just barely yields to horsewhip and goad combined."[18] The charioteer and the good horse must work together to tame and curb the willfulness of the dark horse, which is

15 Plato, *Phaedr.*, 246a–b.
16 Ibid., 247b.
17 Ibid., 247d.
18 Ibid., 253d–e.

prone to pursue its own direction and difficult to correct. They must batter and bloody it whenever it veers from the proper course, until it learns to submit to authority. Only through severe discipline can its insolence be broken. If this is done properly, then when this horse confronts something for which it lusts, it is too fearful to engage in pursuit.

This is a portrait of the human soul, in which reason and passion undergo a perpetual dialectical struggle for dominance. To attain the good life, rational judgment must assess which goods are truly beneficial, and self-control is needed for the pursuit of these worthy goods. The Dionysian impulses are always present, and always threaten to overturn the carriage, or to sink it from the heights of bliss into the earthy mud. Properly trained and held in check, they can do great work in pulling the load. However, where this discipline breaks down, the danger always lurks that in a sudden passion it will guide the entire cart off a precipice.

Aschenbach becomes the victim of the irrational guidance of the dark horse. His charioteer nods, and the result is a series of ignoble decisions that result in his needless death. The temptation in pandemic times may be to give the dark horse run of the chariot. This is what the rational faculty must avoid at all costs. In the present crisis, it is not statistically likely that submission to Dionysian impulses will result in our deaths. However, it necessarily results in a loss of dignity, and a ridiculousness and unseemliness that are always imprudent. It distances one from the good life and right action. Dionysus tamed is a great boon, but Dionysus unleashed turns respectable men and women into grotesques.

CHAPTER VIII

Albert Camus

The Plague

Practice Common Decency

Albert Camus (1913–60) was a writer in many fields—philosopher, playwright, journalist—but his finest works were the handful of novels he produced in his short life. Camus received the Nobel Prize for Literature in 1957 "for his important literary production, which with clear-sighted earnestness illuminates the problems of the human conscience in our times."[1] *The Stranger*, a story about Meursault, a young French Algerian who indifferently kills an Arab and is later executed, remains a favorite amongst college undergraduates. *The Fall*, an existential reflection about the fall of man, was called by Jean-Paul Sartre "perhaps the finest and least understood" of his books.[2] The most ambitious of Camus' works, however, is his 1947 novel *The Plague* (*La Peste*), in which Camus explores his usual existential themes with reference not to an individual, but an entire community. Because it chronicles the sudden outbreak of plague in the Algerian city of Oran, *The Plague* is also Camus' most resonant novel in the age of COVID-19.

Camus' contemporary, the philosopher Maurice Merleau-Ponty, once wrote, "The work of a great novelist always rests on two or three philosophical ideas. For Stendhal, these are the notions of the Ego and Liberty; for Balzac, the mystery of history as the appearance of a meaning in chance events; for Proust, the way the past is involved in the present and the presence of times gone by. The function of the novelist is not to state these ideas thematically but to make them exist for us in the way that things exist."[3] If this is not universally true, it is at least often the case. The novelist interprets the world in a certain way and that mode of understanding permeates his or her works. The more deeply the author has struggled over

1 "The Nobel Prize in Literature 1957." NobelPrize.org. Nobel Media AB 2020. Wed. 24 Jun 2020. Accessible at: https://www.nobelprize.org/prizes/literature/1957/summary/.

2 Jean-Paul Sartre, "Tribute to Albert Camus," in *Camus: A Collection of Critical Essays*, ed. Germaine Brée (Englewood Cliffs, NJ: Prentice-Hall, 1962), 173.

3 Maurice Merleau-Ponty, "Metaphysics and the Novel," in *Sense and Non-Sense*, trans. Hubert L. Dreyfus and Patricia Allen Dreyfus (Evanston, IL: Northwestern University Press, 1964), 26.

a few metaphysical questions, the more thoroughly these ideas permeate every book. Each literary production is, in a sense, a partial answer to these questions. The regularity of these central ideas allows us to use the names of great authors as adjectives; it is proper to call a situation "Dickensian" or "Proustian," for example.

Camus's work (both fiction and non-fiction) is permeated by a single philosophical problem. The clarity that he gives to this problem and the courage with which he confronts it without blinking give his work its power. Camus articulates the problem in his philosophical essay, "The Myth of Sisyphus," where he writes, "This world in itself is not reasonable, that is all that can be said. What is absurd is the confrontation of this irrational [universe] and the wild longing for clarity whose call echoes in the human heart."[4] The reality of the universe is chaos and incoherence. The paradox of human existence is the perpetual conflict between the inherently senseless world and the human need for sense and order. Camus refers to this psychological longing as the *nostalgia for unity*. He writes, "That nostalgia for unity, that appetite for the absolute illustrates the essential impulse of the human drama. But the fact of that nostalgia's existence does not imply that it is to be immediately satisfied."[5] The nostalgic agent forever yearns for coherence in existence, and this coherence is never forthcoming. For Camus, the world does not inherently make sense of follow any script, yet we cannot help looking for the sense in things. Since this irreconcilable dialectic is at play at all times, the character of the world is fundamentally *absurd*. Sisyphus is the personification of the absurdity of existence, endlessly pushing his boulder up a mountain only to see it roll back again when he reaches the top. We must ever look for meaning, and we are doomed to failure. The very act of living, Camus says, "is keeping absurdity alive."[6]

The theme of the absurdity of life, specifically in reference to the unending conflict between the search for order and the reality of chaos, is the metaphysical idea at the core of all of Camus' writing. He has no *argument* that existence is essentially absurd, and he offers no proofs or deductions. We as readers are free to accept or reject his worldview, insofar as it resonates with our own experience. This is his weakness as a philosopher. At the same time, his aptitude for transforming this idea into

4 Albert Camus, "The Myth of Sisyphus," in *The Myth of Sisyphus and Other Essays*, trans. Justin O'Brien (New York: Vintage, 1955), 16.

5 Ibid., 13.

6 Ibid., 40.

imagery and narrative is his strength as a novelist. Merleau-Ponty writes that "existential philosophy assigns itself the task, not of explaining the world or of discovering its 'conditions of possibility,' but rather of formulating an experience of the world, a contact with the world which precedes all thought *about* the world."[7] For Merleau-Ponty, the tasks of existential philosophy and literature are one and the same, namely the presentation of experience. Camus' writing is therefore a living portrait of the absurd. On a deeper level, we must also remain aware that the absurd cannot be represented in language. The root of "absurd" is the Latin *surdus* (mute), and the mathematical "surd" is an irrational number. The absurd can neither be spoken nor written. If literature attempts to portray absurdity, this task is doomed in advance to futility. Camus' novels are Sisyphean labors through and through.

Recognition of the meaninglessness of life can lead to crushing despair, as we will see with Ingmar Bergman's hero, Antonius Block. "The Myth of Sisyphus" begins from the dark question of whether suicide is an appropriate response to the discovery of meaninglessness. Camus counsels, however, that suicide is not an acceptable solution to life's absurdity. It is only acceptance of the essential absurdity of life that can yield victory. Human dignity, and even heroism, arises when the individual admits the meaninglessness of existence and continues on anyway. Doomed to failure, the human spirit may still choose to go forward regardless. Great works of absurdity are always tragicomedies because of this dual character. The spirit of the tragicomic is captured the final line of Samuel Beckett's *Molloy* trilogy: "I can't go on, I'll go on."[8] Sisyphus is such a character. He knows his labor will never end, and yet he continues the effort anyway. Camus writes, "The struggle itself toward the heights is enough to fill a man's heart. One must imagine Sisyphus happy."[9] Likewise, Meursault finds peace at the end of *The Stranger* by accepting life's absurdity. In spite of the meaninglessness of his short life, he affirms while awaiting execution, "I felt that I had been happy and that I was happy again."[10]

The Plague is a masterpiece of absurdity. The plague itself is the very image of absurdity, killing and devastating the population of Oran without meaning or moral. For Camus, there is no response to the plague that is

---

7 Merleau-Ponty, "Metaphysics," 27-28.

8 Samuel Beckett, *The Unnamable*, in *Three Novels* (New York: Grove Weidenfeld, 1991), 414.

9 Camus, "Myth of Sisyphus," 91.

10 Albert Camus, *The Stranger*, trans. Matthew Ward (New York: Vintage, 1989), 123.

not equally groundless. A new generation of readers is currently discovering this book, as it has been recently recommended as necessary quarantine reading by the *New York Times*, *Los Angeles Times*, *Washington Post*, Al Jazeera, the BBC, and most other major media sources throughout the world.[11] Primary school teachers have been assigning the book to quarantined students. Those familiar with the book of old are revisiting it as a prophetic manual of sorts. *The Plague* has suddenly entered the bestseller lists of several nations, and it has been the work of plague literature that has benefitted most from COVID-19. There is no need to argue for its importance today, since the free market has already decided the question.

The Plague is set in Camus' native Algeria. He was born in Bondavi to French parents during World War I. After his father was killed at the battle of the Marne, Camus was raised by his deaf mother in a low-income neighborhood in Algiers. He belonged to several communist organizations as a young man and wrote for the left-wing newspaper *Alger républican* during the years that saw the rise of fascism and Nazism in Europe. In the 1940s, Camus lived in Paris, where he actively worked for the French Resistance during the Nazi occupation of France, writing and editing for the resistance newspaper *Combat*. Tuberculosis would compel Camus to reside in France for most of the remainder of his life, but Algeria remained the inspiration and setting for much of his writing. The city of Oran, where *The Plague* takes place, was Camus' home for a time in 1940. His relationship to the location was mixed. Even though it provided inspiration for the setting and plot of *The Stranger*, Camus often "stewed about the lack of cultural life in Oran," and denounced its "provincialism."[12] In the opening paragraph of *The Plague*, Camus writes that "everyone agreed," given the extraordinary nature of the events in the book, "they were out of place [in Oran]" (3).[13]

Oran has had a long history of medical epidemics. As a port city situated on the Mediterranean Sea, Oran has the same vulnerability to contagion as the Italian port cities that were so frequently ravaged by plague. The intermingling of persons and cargoes from three continents repeatedly

11 See, for example, Alain de Botton, "Camus on the Coronavirus," *The New York Times* (19 Mar. 2020); Stephen Metcalf, "Albert Camus' 'The Plague' and our own Great Reset," *Los Angeles Times* (23 Mar. 2020); and Roger Lowenstein, "In Camus' 'The Plague,' lessons about fear, quarantine and the human spirit," *The Washington Post* (3 Apr. 2020).

12 Olivier Todd, *Albert Camus: A Life* (New York: Carroll & Graf, 2000), 99.

13 All parenthetical citations in this section refer to Albert Camus, *The Plague*, trans. Stuart Gilbert (New York: Modern Library, 1948).

introduced disease to the region and hastened its spread. Oran was struck by bubonic plague as early as the fourteenth century, and suffered serious outbreaks in 1556 and 1678. Minor outbreaks recurred into the mid-twentieth century, with cases reported as late as 1946, the year before Camus published *The Plague*. An outbreak of eighteen cases of plague surprisingly arose in the summer of 2003 after decades without a case.[14] More relevant to the composition of Camus' novel was the severe 1849 cholera epidemic that claimed three thousand lives in Oran. This outbreak is thought to have been the inspiration for *The Plague*, though the events of the novel are set in the 1940s.[15] The plague that is at the center of Camus' narrative was not, however, a historical event. It was entirely an invention of the literary imagination.

As a plot device, the plague serves the function of placing the novel's characters under extreme duress, in order to analyze their behavior and emotional responses. The psyche under duress is a favorite trope of existential literature, from Dostoevsky's epic novels to James Dickey's *Deliverance*. Everyday behavior, with its low stakes, requires little prudence. Under extreme circumstances, everyday behavior ceases to yield the desired results. War is such a circumstance, as is a deadly epidemic. New, unfamiliar rules of right action must be learned. These conditions force us to examine more closely what is demanded by prudential wisdom.

The Plague is rich in psychological insight and symbolism. The story is narrated by Dr. Bernard Rieux, an atheist whose wife is an inpatient at a sanitarium. The narrator is anonymous for most of the book, and Rieux only reveals himself in the final few pages. He justifies this anonymity as necessary for "adopting the tone of an impartial observer" (271). The epidemic begins with the outbreak of an undiagnosed plight that kills an extraordinary number of rats in Oran. Shortly thereafter, Dr. Rieux treats an elderly patient who presents a number of symptoms: "He had started feeling pains all over—in his neck, armpits, and groin," and in his neck, "a hard lump, like a knot in wood, had formed" (16). Later, the symptoms advance to include "vomiting pinkish bile," a high-grade fever, internal pains, and the appearance of black patches on the thighs (19). A few days later the old man dies in feverish agony. Rieux hears of other patients suffering from an undiagnosed illness with the same general pathology. Finally, he is forced to conclude the inconvenient truth: "It's hardly credible.

---

14 Eric Bertherat et al, "Plague Reappearance in Algeria after 50 Years, 2003," *Emerging Infectious Diseases* 13 (Oct. 2007): 1459–62.

15 Peta Mitchell, *Contagious Metaphor* (New York: Bloomsbury, 2014), 50.

But everything points to its being plague" (33).

From this slow beginning, the plague begins to spread rapidly through the city. A pest-house is established, which is quickly filled to capacity with the infected. A small quantity of plague serum arrives, but this is insufficient to meet the needs of the population and is soon depleted. Government is slow to act, with local officials deferring any decisive action until orders come from above. Finally, with dozens of people dying every day, administrators are compelled to admit a plague outbreak and seal off the town. Communication with the outside world is drastically limited, and there is no passage in or out of the city gates. Camus writes, "Plague had killed all colors, vetoed pleasure" (104). Rieux, an idealistic vacationer named Jean Tarrou, and a civil clerk named Joseph Grand lead the efforts to treat the disease as it spreads, recruiting many volunteer workers for the purpose. As conditions in the town deteriorate, the "prisoners of plague" (151) become more and more despondent. Escape attempts are made, but the escapees are shot by sentries. Violence and petty crime increase, leading to the declaration of martial law. Victims of the plague are promptly cremated without ceremony. Hope is renounced, as there is no cure in sight and no exit from the hellish town. The spirit of the people of Oran wastes away in the emotionally numbing "sound of a huge concourse of people marking time, a never ending, stifling drone that, gradually swelling, filled the town from end to end, and evening after evening gave its truest, mournfulest expression to the blind endurance that had ousted love from all our hearts" (168).

In the autumn, Grand is stricken with the plague and declines to the point of death. However, he surprisingly recovers overnight, and Rieux is shocked by this "resurrection" (239). This marks the beginning of a trend, as other patients likewise miraculously recover. Soon, rats are once again out in the streets for the first time since the outbreak began, and mortality figures finally begin to decrease. As winter progresses, the plague goes into dramatic decline. Historically, pandemics have tended to end in this way, the root disease becoming less and less deadly without warning or human melioration. For Camus, there is as much meaninglessness in the end of the plague as in its beginning. The town reopens and lovers are reunited. However, even amidst this success, the disease still manages to claim a few final victims, the idealist Tarrou among them.

Camus reflects on the senselessness of all of this for both the survivors and the dead: "Tarrou had 'lost the match,' as he put it. But what had he, Rieux, won? No more than the experience of having known plague and remembering it, of having known friendship and remembering it, of knowing affection and being destined to one day remember it" (262). For Camus, this is the absurdity of the human condition. There is no higher meaning in human experience, which is finally reducible to a mere handful of memories. However, Rieux, like Sisyphus and Meursault, reaffirms existence by praising the people who admit this absurdity while nevertheless acting decently. He says, "Dr. Rieux resolved to compile this chronicle, so that he should not be one of those who hold their peace but should bear witness in favor of those plague-stricken people; so that some memorial of the injustice and outrage done them might endure; and to state quite simply what we learn in a time of pestilence: that there are more things to admire in men than to despise" (278).

This positive note at the book's conclusion summarizes the main idea of the book. Though life is absurd, and the universe works without meaning or order, it is always within one's power to choose to do one's duty. Dr. Rieux continues to do his duty as the world crumbles around him. Every day, he continues to treat as many patients as he can, both in hospitals and in his own home. He does not cavil and he does not retreat in from the infected. He is aware that the amount of exposure he opens himself to is likely to end in his own death, and he is likewise aware that he is powerless to prevent the suffering and demise of his patients. His labors are bound to fail. He faces these truths not with the desperate hopefulness of Samuel Beckett's heroes, but with tough-minded clarity. Nevertheless, he goes on doing as much as he is able. At one point, a journalist named Rambert presses Rieux on the fruitlessness of his work. Rambert says, "You haven't understood that [the plague] means exactly that—the same thing over and over and over again" (148). The doctor is rolling boulders up a hill, toward an apex he can never reach. Rambert suggests that Rieux perhaps hungers for heroism, which the doctor denies. Rieux says, "There's one thing I must tell you: there's no question of heroism in all this. It's a matter of common decency. That's an idea which may make some people smile, but the only means of fighting a plague is—common decency" (150).

Common decency is the great lesson of *The Plague*. Camus' counsel for right action in a pandemic is reducible to these three words: *practice common decency*. "What do you mean by common decency?" asks Rambert. "I don't know what it means for other people," Rieux responds. "But for me it consists in doing my job" (150). What exactly *is* common decency? This term has no universally recognized meaning. However, it is neither empty verbiage nor a sloppy use of language. It is the correct term to use if existence itself is likewise without meaning. Common decency is determined by one's moral sense, and is synonymous with the word "ought." To behave decently is to do what we ought to do, and this is determined in each individual by a complex web of circumstances and relationships. Rieux is a practical, analytical man, and his "common decency" is nothing metaphysical or spiritually elevated. It is the pragmatic imperative to fulfill the duties of his station. He is a physician, and physicians treat the sick. Rieux's morality is rooted in concrete existence, not philosophy. "A man can't cure and know at the same time," he says. "So let's cure as quickly as we can. That's the more urgent job" (189).

This practical human decency is the most rational form of morality for one who accepts the doctrine of absurdism and has no belief in the divine. The atheist always stumbles over the problem of how moral principles can be constructed if existence is inherently chaotic. For the religious mentality, the divine transmits the code of right action to the human world, either directly or indirectly, and this code is sanctified by omnipotence. Even the deist is able to tie morality to reason in history. However, without God as the guarantor of morality, absolute moral relativism becomes the obstacle with which ethical thinkers must contend. If there is no meaning, then on what grounds is anything right or wrong? The proclamation of Hamlet, "There is nothing either good or bad but thinking makes it so,"[16] is then at least plausible. Camus' Caligula poses the central question of the atheistic moralist: "Who can condemn me in this world where there is no judge, where nobody is innocent?"[17]

Dr. Rieux is an atheist, and he has no illusions about his actions winning him favor in an eternal beyond. Asked by Tarrou if he believes in God, Rieux answers, "No—but what does that really mean? I'm fumbling in the dark, trying to make something out. But I've long ceased to find that original." This irreligion gives him the motive for his calling. He says that, were he to believe in Providence, "he would cease curing the sick and leave that to Him" (116). In Rieux's view, the calling of the physician is to "struggle with all our might against death, without raising our eyes toward the heaven where He sits in silence." Tarrou counters, "But your victories will never be lasting." "Yes, I know that," says Rieux. "But it's no

---

16 William Shakespeare, *Hamlet*, in *The Oxford Shakespeare*, ed. John Jowett et al (New York: Oxford University Press, 2005), II.ii.251-52.

17 Albert Camus, *Caligula*, in *Caligula and 3 Other Plays*, trans. Stuart Gilbert (New York: Random House, 1958), 72.

reason for giving up the struggle." He admits that the plague is a "never ending defeat," but he is not discouraged. He says that his preceptor for this worldview has been "suffering" (118).

The most concise statement about existentialist ethics was given by Sartre, Camus' friend and collaborator. In his essay "Existentialism is a Humanism," Sartre describes an occasion on which a student approached him for advice. The young man was torn between two courses of action during the time of the Nazi occupation of France. He could stay at home to support his mother, as he was her only surviving child and only source of consolation. Or he could leave for England and serve in the Free French Forces, fighting for the liberty of his homeland. To choose the former would be to the detriment of his country, but to choose the latter would leave his mother in despair. Neither deontological nor utilitarian ethics can give a convincing solution to such a dilemma, in which the individual, like Antigone, is torn between equally pressing obligations. The answer that Sartre gives is the only answer a wise man can offer: "You're free, choose, that is, invent. No general ethics can tell you what is to be done; there are no omens in the world. The Catholics will reply, 'But there are.' Granted—but, in any case, I myself choose the meaning they have."[18] For Sartre, there is no better or worse choice. The ethically important thing is to make *some* choice, whatever it may be, and keep to it.

Dr. Rieux chooses to fulfill his professional station, and to treat those with disease, even at the risk of death. This, for him, is the demand of common decency, the demand of the "ought." Nevertheless, he recognizes that common decency may have different meanings to other individuals. As Rieux affirms, there are many characters in *The Plague* who are admirable, even though they are not all driven by the same motives. Tarrou, for example, despite being a visitor in Oran, puts all of his efforts into hopelessly fighting the plague, even unto his own pointless death. He is an idealist, motivated by lofty principles. When Dr. Rieux directly interrogates him on his reasons for taking a leading hand in the struggle, Tarrou responds, "I don't know. My code of morals, perhaps." "Your code of morals? What code?" "Comprehension" (120). This cryptic answer suggests the understanding that the plague is the equal responsibility of all, just as all citizens are responsible for the atrocities of their governments. Later, he tells Rieux, "It comes to this, what interests me is learning how to become a saint" (230). Since Tarrou too is an atheist, his dilemma is the

18 Jean-Paul Sartre, *Existentialism and Human Emotions*, trans. Hazel E. Barnes and Bernard Frechtman (New York: Philosophical Library, 1957), 24–28.

question of how to become a saint in the absence of God. This is an absurd dilemma, containing an irreconcilable paradox. Whatever Tarrou's ideals, though, the result is the same as Rieux's pragmatic sensibilities: common decency.

Other characters respond to the plague in other fashions. Joseph Grand is an unassuming civil servant who takes up oversight of the complicated logistics of the medical efforts to fight the plague. He has nothing of the hero about him, but places himself in a thankless position of great responsibility. Rieux calls him "the true embodiment of the quiet courage that inspired the sanitary groups. He said yes without a moment's hesitation and with the large-heartedness that was a second nature to him" (123). Father Paneloux is a Jesuit priest in the town, who aids the medical efforts while seeing the plague as a test of faith. "My brothers," he preaches, "a time of testing has come for us all. We must believe everything or deny everything. And who among you would dare to deny everything?" (202). In the face of an absurd reality, one option is always the abandonment of reason and the acceptance of the will of God. This is the position of Kierkegaard, who writes, "When I let go of the demonstration, the existence is there. ... This diminutive moment, however brief it is—it does not have to be long, because it is a leap."[19] This leap of faith entails the suspension of rational demonstration, and the ungrounded affirmation of transcendental order. Still others in the town have other responses to the crisis. Even as crime began to rise, "the Cathedral was practically always full of worshippers" (86), as religion becomes a source of consolation for many. Other "fledgling moralists" went around "proclaiming there was nothing to be done about it and we should bow to the inevitable" (122).

All of these positions arise from different temperaments—some humble, some noble; some atheistic, some theistic—but, for Camus, none is ultimately best. "Common decency" is not the possession of one particular type of individual. Every decision is a moral decision, as Sartre says. The meaningful thing is not the content of the decision, but the extent to which one resolutely follows through. What are we to do when, as Thomas Flynn says, "we long for meaning conveyed by a Universe that cares but discover only an empty sky"?[20] We can only choose to do our best, in keeping with our station in society, and to perform our duty. The choice to

19 Søren Kierkegaard, *Philosophical Fragments*, trans. Howard V. Hong and Edna H. Hong (Princeton, NJ: Princeton University Press, 1985), 43.

20 Thomas R. Flynn, *Existentialism: A Very Short Introduction* (New York: Oxford University Press, 2006), 47.

do so is itself absurd, since it is ungrounded. We could just as well choose to shirk our duty, so long as we spent our lives reaffirming that decision every day. However, to do so would be to make the world worse. For the absurdist, the ethics of common decency might not be acceptable to everyone. However, it is the decision that transforms the tragedy of life into a tragicomedy and produces a smile on the face of Sisyphus.

Common decency has one ruling principle: *make no one's life the worse for having known you.* To choose the path of decency is, in the end, just as futile as any other path. All paths lead to the grave. However, decency is what makes suffering bearable. The selfless, thankless efforts of Rieux, Tassou, and company do not defeat the plague in Oran, but they do improve the conditions of some individuals for some amount of time. To do one's duty in Camus' sense is to take responsibility for the misfortune of one's fellow human beings. To make this decision yields little that is tangible. As Rieux says, all that remains is a memory of friendship, a memory of the plague, and scarce anything else. However, it also makes life more tolerable for some, and it makes life the worse for none. This is the spiritual victory of the tragicomedian.

The Plague has often been read as an allegory for the French Resistance during occupation. His commentator, Germaine Brée, writes that historical chance presented Camus with "the sinister universe of the second world war, a real universe of arbitrary mass-murder and execution in the name of necessity or ideology, the stifling world of enemy occupation and tyranny,"[21] and that Camus transformed this concrete universe into his beleaguered Oran. Resistance to tyranny, like resistance to a medical outbreak, is a slow and thankless job, one that requires the small labors of many men and women every day. For this reason, *The Plague* serves as a moral lesson for all times of crisis. Brée observes, "The undramatic and stubborn fight Rieux and his friends organize against the Plague, their human refusal to submit to its domination are presented as the record, not of a theory, nor of a faith, but of an experience. … The reader draws from the book a sense of human dignity and probity to which he cannot help responding."[22] The resistance offered by the heroes of *The Plague* is certainly undramatic, and the book has nothing of the Homeric about it. This lack is intentional, as it is in the work of Thomas Mann. A pandemic is not an evil that can be vanquished through a single heroic action. It is an evil that must be fought with patience, compassion, and small acts of decency.

---

21 Germaine Brée, "Albert Camus and the Plague," *Yale French Studies* 8 (1951): 98.
22 Ibid., 99.

The task of common decency is not the glorious self-sacrifice of Achilles, which even the gods behold with admiration. It is an everyday decision to do what one can.

Camus' "common decency" is the single most important mandate of prudence during the COVID-19 pandemic. The practice day in and day out of decency is what keeps a suffering people from complete spiritual atrophy. What this means for each of us is different, and depends upon our own unique situation. If you are a nurse, it is your duty to nurse. If you are a philosopher, philosophize. If you have children, see to their well-being and education every day. If you are without family, do what you can to help your community. If you have elderly people in your household, resist the urge to take an active hand in public works. If you have access to supplies that are needed, make them available. If you are a person of the cloth, comfort others with the Word of God. Whatever you are, be that thing; decency has no universal manual.

Why should we choose to practice common decency and do our duty? This, for Camus, is one more absurd question. It is possible—even likely—that our small, persistent acts of good faith will have no impact whatsoever in the outcome of this crisis. This futility is all too clear today to far too many. However, as Dr. Rieux says, this is no reason to give up the struggle. It is needful that we continue every day to try, like Sisyphus, to reach the top of the hill. To abandon your station is to accept that people's lives may be worse for having known you. This is to renounce human dignity. If we wish to engage in the losing game of existence, we are obligated to try to win. Such is the very character of the human condition. This quixotic, paradoxical lesson is the single insight that Camus offered to the world. To act morally in a meaningless world without gods, we must act so as to preserve human dignity, doing what we can if only *because* we can.

CHAPTER IX

Ingmar Bergman

The Seventh Seal

Redeem the World by the Charitable Deed

The word "literature" is derived from the Latin *littera*, letter of the alphabet. In common usage, "literature" usually refers only to books or other written works. Insofar as cinema makes use of the spoken word as its medium, and it is usually the staged performance of a written script, there is a sense in which a film could be called a work of literature. However, this usage is unusual and reductive. Along with its connection to language, film has additional functions that have nothing to do with the written word, such as the establishment of what Walter Benjamin calls "equilibrium between human beings and the [mechanical] apparatus."[1] A more compelling argument is possible for the claim that literature and cinema are both species of poetry. As mentioned in the introduction, the word "poetry" is derived from the Greek ποίησις (*poiesis*). *Poiesis* is an action by which something is brought into being. It is an act of spiritual creation. In Plato's *Symposium*, the priestess Diotima says that *poiesis* consists of being "pregnant in soul—because there surely *are* those who are even more pregnant in their souls than in their bodies, and these are pregnant with what is fitting for a soul to bear and bring to birth. And what is fitting? Wisdom and the rest of virtue, which all poets beget."[2] Any artist who transforms brute matter through imaginative spiritual activity is a poet.

Without introducing a digression on what constitutes "art," we may say that at least some films are genuine artistic achievements. Great films are works of *poiesis*, and they bear comparison to literature, a sister form of poetry. As Marshall McLuhan says, "It would be difficult to exaggerate the bond between print and movie in terms of their power to generate fantasy in the viewer or reader."[3] The movie and the book both aim to pull the

1 Walter Benjamin, "The Work of Art in the Age of Its Technological Reproducibility," in *The Work of Art in the Age of Its Technological Reproducibility and Other Writings on Media*, trans. Edmund Jephcott et al. (Cambridge, MA: Belknap Press, 2008), 37.

2 Plato, *Symp.*, 209a.

3 Marshall McLuhan, *Understanding Media: The Extensions of Man* (New York: Signet, 1966), 249.

audience into an imaginary world through the mediation of *Logos*, the word.

To write a book about plague literature that rigorously binds itself to the written word is folly when a film concerning plague exists that is a true masterpiece of *poiesis*. Such a film is the 1957 Swedish classic *The Seventh Seal* (*Det sjunde inseglet*), written and directed by Ingmar Bergman (1918–2007). *The Seventh Seal* is a beautiful parable about the absence of God and the search for meaning. It is closer to the morality plays of the late Middle Ages than the computer-generated fantasies that have replaced story-telling in film today. If its dialogue and imagery feel heavy-handed at times, that is a condemnation of our modern superficiality rather than a shortcoming of the film. *The Seventh Seal* is an artwork created for meditative human beings, not the technological person of today. The film critic Roger Ebert writes, "Films are no longer concerned with the silence of God, but with the chattering of men. We are uneasy to find Bergman asking existential questions in an age of irony. ... But the directness of *The Seventh Seal* is its strength: This is an uncompromising film, regarding good and evil with the same simplicity and faith as its hero."[4]

The Seventh Seal began as a short play that Bergman wrote for his drama students in 1952–53, titled *Wood Painting*. In his autobiography, Bergman says that *Wood Painting* transformed into *The Seventh Seal* "under difficult circumstances in a surge of vitality and delight." The ideas and images of the film evolved out of Bergman's obsession with the visual imagery of medieval Swedish churches. The *Seventh Seal* has the feel of a monastic fresco put into movement and caught on film. Bergman writes, "Like all churchgoers at all times, I have often become lost in altar pieces, triptychs, crucifixes, stained glass windows in murals." In these pious representations, Bergman found "the Knight playing chess with Death. Death sawing down the Tree of Life, a terrified wretch wringing his hands at the top. Death leading the dance to the Dark Lands, wielding his scythe like a flag, the congregation capering in a long line and the jester bringing up the rear."[5] The entire movie was shot in just thirty-five days, with a budget of $150,000.[6]

The plot of *The Seventh Seal* is simple and straightforward, after the fashion of medieval drama. A knight and his squire return home from war

---

4 Roger Ebert, "The Seventh Seal," in *The Great Movies* (New York: Broadway Books, 2002), 405–6.

5 Ingmar Bergman, *The Magic Lantern: An Autobiography*, trans. Joan Tate (Chicago: University of Chicago Press, 2007), 273–74.

6 Melvyn Bragg, *The Seventh Seal* (London: British Film Institute, 1993), 48.

to find their land ravaged by the Black Death. The knight encounters Death personified and challenges the specter to a game of chess, with the understanding that he will remain alive as long as the game continues. As the knight and squire journey homeward to the knight's castle, they encounter various characters in search of their own meaning, some of whom travel along with the knight. Death follows and is present everywhere, reaping without interest or bias. The knight and his party venture through a silent wood, and finally reach the castle, which is the goal of their quest. There they meet Death, who has won the game, and all succumb except for a family of thespians who escape through the cleverness of the knight. The whole of the plot is foretold from the start, for Death cannot lose. The plague will consume everything in the end.

At play in this narrative are many of the traditional archetypes of psychology. Archetypes are basic symbols, the significances of which are universally recognized. Carl Jung defines archetypes as "the contents of the collective unconscious."[7] In *The Seventh Seal*, it is not just a few that are present, but they abound in every scene. The entire film is a Heroic Quest; the knight's castle is the Promised Land; the chess game is the Magic Key. Death is the Trickster, and his subterfuge in the chess game is the Dirty Trick. Jons is the Charming Scoundrel; the girl he rescues is the Damsel in Distress; the rogue ex-priest Raval is the Barbarian. The whole of the barren country, where Block and Jons return after the Holy War, is Purgatory.[8] All of these ideas are familiar and their significance is immediately understood from our own dreams. Because we know them so well, the plot carries little suspense.

However, the plot is only secondary and, as with all poetic dramas, serves primarily as a vehicle for ideas. The strength and terrible beauty of the movie is its exploration of existential doubt and the relationship of life to mortality. The title of the movie is derived from the Book of Revelation, and references the end of the world. The Revelator says, "When the Lamb opened the seventh seal, there was silence in heaven for about half an hour. And I saw the seven angels who stand before God, and seven trumpets were given to them."[9] Silence is one of the central motifs in the movie. Silence and stillness are used for dramatic effect in various scenes, and

7 Carl Jung, *The Archetypes and the Collective Unconscious*, trans. R. F. C. Hull (Princeton, NJ: Princeton University Press, 1990), 4.

8 Umberto Eco gives a similar analysis of the use of archetypes in *Casablanca*. See "Casablanca: Cult Movies and Intertextual Collage," in *Travels in Hyperreality*, trans. William Weaver (New York: Harcourt Brace & Company, 1986), esp. 202–9.

9 Rev. 8:1-2.

Bergman's use of silence is far more eloquent than speech. The knight Antonius Block (played to perfection by an ashen Max von Sydow) sends his squire Jons (Gunnar Björnstrand) to ask directions from what turns out to be a rotting corpse, its eyes burrowed out of the skull. Jons tells his master, "He was quite eloquent. ... The trouble is that what he had to say was most depressing" (4).[10] A nameless girl rescued early in the film by Jons is the personification of eloquent silence. She speaks only four lines in the movie, but is far more perceptive and empathetic than the characters who bide their time with idle chatter. On a higher level, the film is an exploration of the silence of God. The plague devastates the human world, while God remains hidden. He does not speak, and His abandoned creation flails about longing for guidance.

Amidst this silence, abandoned by God, the knight Antonius Block returns to his home land disillusioned from ten years fighting in the Crusades. Block is Job in Quixote's armor. As the film opens, he awakens on a barren and stony beach, his squire Jons still asleep. A ghastly figure robed in black with a powdered white face, his hands hidden in his cloak, stands behind Block. This figure is Death. Though they have not met directly, Death has been beside Block for the last ten years, as the knight has had to kill in the name of God and watch many comrades killed in turn, in the name of a different God. "I have been walking by your side for a long time," says Death. Block replies, "That I know." The knight is not afraid to die, since he has long since lost all pleasure with life. Nevertheless, he stalls Death by suggesting a game of chess. Death accepts the challenge, but asks why Block wants to play the game with him. "I have my reasons," says Block (2). Throughout the film, the pair revisit their chess game repeatedly, with fortune tilting now in one direction, now the other.

We discover Block's purpose in forestalling his own death when he confesses to Death in the guise of a priest. Block says, "My heart is empty. The emptiness is a mirror turned towards my face. I see myself in it, and I am filled with fear and disgust. Through my indifference to my fellow men, I have isolated myself from their company. Now I live in a world of phantoms. I am imprisoned in my dreams and fantasies." "And yet you don't want to die?" Death asks. "Yes, I do." "What are you waiting for?" "I want knowledge" (11–12). The knowledge that Block desires is

---

10 All parenthetical citations in this section refer to the film *The Seventh Seal* [*Det sjunde inseglet*], dir. Ingmar Bergman (Stockholm: Svensk Filmindustri, 1957). For page numbers, see the translated transcript of the film, accessible at: http://www.astro.puc.cl/~rparra/tools/ROCK_EDITIONS/det_sjunde_inseglet.pdf.

certainty about the existence of God. His existential dread stems from the absence of a God that will not manifest Himself. "I want knowledge, not faith, not suppositions, but knowledge. I want God to stretch out His hand towards me, reveal Himself and speak to me." When Block calls out, no one answers, and no one seems to be there. If there is no God, "Then life is an outrageous horror. No one can live in the face of death, knowing that all is nothingness" (13).

Block's youthful piety was abused by a charlatan priest, who exploited his innocence to inspire a passion for a meaningless and godless war. Now Block faces the crisis of faith that Miguel de Unamuno says gives rise to the tragic sense of life. Unamuno writes, "The most tragic problem of philosophy is to reconcile intellectual necessities with the necessities of the heart and the will. For it is on this rock that every philosophy that pretends to resolve the eternal and tragic contradiction, the basis of our existence, breaks to pieces. But do all men face this contradiction squarely?"[11] The heart hungers for belief in a beyond, while the intellect knows that certainty about God is impossible. Knowledge and faith are irreconcilable. Most people do *not* dare to squarely confront this problem, and prefer to lose themselves in the sports pages and the idle gossip of streetcorners. To confront the contradiction of reason and faith is almost a heroic act. Nietzsche warns, "When you look long into an abyss, the abyss looks into you."[12] Consorting too long with nothingness has consequences for one's inner life.

Since his intellect cannot avoid the tragic recognition that certainty of God is not forthcoming, Block has a practical project that he hopes will give meaning or value to his life at its end. Halfway between life and death, being and nothing, Block tells his confessor, "My life has been a futile pursuit, a wandering, a great deal of talk without meaning. I feel no bitterness or self-reproach because the lives of most people are very much like this. But I will use my reprieve for one meaningful deed" (13). For Block to perform a meaningful deed, he must create meaning. If God will not speak, then the universe is chaos, nothing more than matter in motion. The human will, however, is capable of creating its own meaning. The very nature of will is meaning-making. The newborn baby is born into a senseless maelstrom of sensations, which William James refers to as "one great

---

11 Miguel de Unamuno, *Tragic Sense of Life*, trans. J. E. Crawford Flitch (New York: Dover, 1954), 15-16.

12 Friedrich Nietzsche, *Beyond Good and Evil*, trans. Walter Kaufmann (New York: Vintage, 1989), §146.

blooming, buzzing confusion."[13] There are blotches of color and sound, but no discreet *things*. From nascence on, the mind carves up the universe into distinct things, fixing identities and imposing patterns on the world. All meaning is made, though seldom consciously. Block—disillusioned and indifferent toward others, both fearless and hopeless—wills to perform one single act that he can consciously invest with significance.

Apart from the aesthetic of Swedish churches and the philosophy of earlier Scandinavian writers (particularly Søren Kierkegaard and August Strindberg), *The Seventh Seal* also shows the influence of medieval religious drama. The allegorical morality play *Everyman*, of unknown authorship, is the best known drama of this type, and similarities can be drawn to Bergman's script. In *Everyman*, the anonymous everyman is approached by Death and told it is time to die. He asks for more time and is refused, but he is allowed to take along one companion. As he prepares for death, he is abandoned by Beauty, Strength, Discretion, and finally even Knowledge. The only companion that follows him into the grave is Good Deeds. Of the personal virtues one carries through life, we are told, "They all at last do every man forsake, / Save his Good Deeds there he doth take."[14] Antonius Block takes up this moral, except that for him God's sanction is not what gives merit to the good deed. He longs to do good *not* for personal redemption, for he has no such illusions, but in order to redeem life itself from the silence of God. The lesson that Bergman teaches us today is that *the charitable deed in times of despair redeems the world.*

As the characters pass through the countryside, being joined by fellow pilgrims all in search of something, they behold the terrors of the plague and the different reactions that others have to the danger. The deeds they see performed are extreme, and aimed at placating a present and angry God. There is nothing world-redeeming or life-affirming about the ritual sacrifices made by the superstitious. These acts cry out for God to redeem the world, which is precisely what Antonius Block is unable to hope for.

Jons is told of the horrors of the plague by a painter before he beholds them himself. The painter explains a ghastly scene he has created: "The remarkable thing is that the poor creatures think the pestilence is the Lord's punishment. Mobs of people who call themselves Slaves of Sin are swarming over the country, flagellating themselves and others, all for the glory of God" (11). Block and Jons later witness such a group of penitents

---

13 William James, *Principles of Psychology*, I:488.

14 A. C. Cawley, ed., *Everyman*, in *Everyman and Medieval Miracle Plays* (New York: E. P. Dutton & Co., 1959), lines 906-7.

engaged in cruel self-torment and humiliation. A theatrical comedy is interrupted by a procession of hooded Dominican monks bearing a large crucified Christ. The monks are followed by a mass of men, women, and children, all bearing whips. The penitents rhythmically flagellate themselves and each other, scourging their own flesh as punishment for the sins of man. They foam at the mouths and twist about in pain; they fall and lift themselves again; they "support each other and help each other to intensify the scourging" (21). They moan in ecstasy, gripped by herd madness. One of the monks chastises the onlookers, "God has sentenced us to punishment. We shall all perish in the black death. ... Death stands right behind you. ... Do you hear the word? You have been sentenced, sentenced!" (21). As the procession passes on its way, some of the broken penitents are unable to continue, but others from the crowd fill their places.

These penitents strive to perform a deed that will redeem the world. However, that deed is misguided. Self-flagellation is an idea conceived in fear, and fear is an irrational passion. Cruel self-torment is the renunciation of the power to act, and presupposes the idea that there is no human meaning in the world. The penitents sacrifice their pleasure and comfort in an attempt to satiate the divine. They assume that only the divine can redeem the human. They view the Black Death as retaliation for the sins of man, and God's silence is a chastisement. In face of this chastisement, the only possible palliative is abnegation and supplication. They beat themselves into a stupor, hoping that this will be enough to coerce God to speak and reinvest the world with meaningfulness. They have nary a thought for redeeming the world themselves.

We encountered this kind of mythical thinking amongst pagans in Thucydides and Christians in Rabelais. We have seen that crisis situations tend to undermine human faith in reason. The individual invests his or her faith in the cult leader, who promises magical solutions for the miseries of the world. In the *Seventh Seal*, monks and priests play the role of shamanistic prophets. The masses embrace the irrational deed out of desperation, lacking faith in the rational deed. Rabelais showed how prophecy hastens the superstitious to ruin by exciting their religious dread. In Roman times, the satirist Lucian criticized those prophets that ruin their flock in the opposite manner, by undermining that dread. He writes, "Many people were over-trustful in the verse [of the false prophet Alexander, promising safety from plague], didn't take precautions, and lived too carelessly ... since they had the words to protect them and unshorn Phoebus to ward off the plague with his arrows."[15] In *The Seventh Seal*, religious dread is turned inward, the affirmation of God's power becomes self-negation, and the organism destroys itself. This deed does not affirm human dignity, but nullifies all meaning in the human world.

Others hypocrites in *The Seventh Seal*, rather than blaming the whole of humankind for the silence of God, invest all of the blame in the iniquities of a single person. The travelers come upon a woman in the stocks with shaved head and an appearance of disorientation. A soldier tells them, "She has had carnal intercourse with the Evil One," and because of this, "she will be burned tomorrow morning at the parish boundary." This *auto da fé* is an expiation offered up to God to appease His wrath. Superstitious minds believe that her suspected liaison with the Devil is the root cause of the plague. A monk warns Block not to speak to her, saying, "She is believed to have caused the pestilence with which we are affected" (15). Later, the pilgrims again encounter this young victim being taken to the place of her execution. After refusing Block's offer of opiates, she tells him that her name is Tyan, and that she is only fourteen years old. Block tells her that he would like to meet the Devil to ask him about God, and she responds that he can, by merely looking into her eyes, as the Devil is always with her. After they stare at one another for some time, the knight turns away in disappointment, and says, "I see fear in your eyes, an empty, numb fear. But nothing else" (42). The pilgrims then watch her burned, and the entire affair is overseen by Death in the likeness of a monk.

The participants of the *auto da fé*—both clerics and laity—hope, by destroying that person so hateful to God, to win back God's love and earn reconciliation to the Holy. These people envision a deed that will save them, but it is a deed of ignorance and wanton cruelty. They are guided as little as the flagellants by reason. They offer up Tyan as a scapegoat for the sins of the world. In Scripture, the scapegoat is an offering made to Yahweh, on whose back are placed the sins of the nation.[16] In *The Seventh Seal*, a touched child stands in for the goat of Leviticus. The violent deed of the zealots redeems nothing. It is itself an act of madness, driven by the irrational terror of hopelessness.

The meaningful deed that Antonius Block finally performs comes from a position not of fear and desperation, but from a place of inner tranquility and decency. Block shows the decency that Camus sanctifies as the

15 Lucian of Samosata, "Alexander or the False Prophet," in *Selected Dialogues*, trans. C. D. N. Costa (New York: Oxford University Press, 2009), 142.

16 Lev. 16:6–10.

one thing needful. Block is well aware of his own pending death. However, in one of his conversations with Death, the latter asks, "Are you going to escort the juggler and his wife through the forest? Those whose names are Jof and Mia and who have a small son?" By this time, this family of performers has taken up with the knight's troop. "Why do you ask?" Block inquires. Death responds, "Oh, no reason at all," and the two look at each other with mutual contempt (35–36). The clear implication is that they too are fated to meet their end, as plague will consume the entire company. These performers, Jof and Mia, are the only characters in the film who are generally content. Their marriage is happy, and they are loving parents of Mikael, a smiling and waddling toddler. The tragic knight's melancholy is only lifted in the presence of the happy family unit. The other members of the company are all seeking redemption of some sort, and they all live beneath the cloud of misfortune and misery. Their choices in life have already damned them. Jof and Mia are also the only fertile characters among the lot. Theirs is the only union that has borne fruit, and Mikael is the symbolic promise of a human future that outlasts the horrid plague.

Seeing his chance, Block uses Death's absorption in the chess game as a distraction whereby Jof and Mia are able to escape from the group with their child. He sacrifices everything on this gambit, as reflected in the game itself. Having earlier in the game given up his knight (self-sacrifice) in order to draw Death into check, he now allows Death to vanquish him entirely. Caught up in the game, Death does not notice Jof, who is himself a visionary, observing the situation and fleeing with his family in their wagon. To keep Death occupied, Block must sacrifice even his queen. Block's wife, to whom we are only introduced once the castle is reached, is among those who are taken by the plague. However, Block must reach the castle with his comrades, and they must all meet their end in order that Death should miss his opportunity and not notice the flight of the performers.

In the end, plague arrives at the castle in the embodiment of Death and the knight, his wife, and his companions are smitten. "[I] welcome you courteously to my house," says Block's wife, and the knight himself bids Death "good morning" (57). Block asks God for mercy, but none among the group complains. In the final scene of the film, Jof and Mia emerge from their wagon after a rainfall, and Mikael crawls on the ground between them. They are safe, preserved by the sacrifice of the others. Jof looks into the distance, where he sees the silhouetted forms of their friends being led off in a dance, with Death at their head and a jester behind. The dance is solemn, but all dance signifies a festival. The abating of the rain and the festival celebration suggest rebirth and a new fertility in the land. The Fisher King is restored. Jof and Mia will survive the plague, but more importantly, the child will survive and the world will continue.

To defeat an opponent at chess is a mark of skill and art. It shows a great technical knowledge and a mastery of strategy. However, prudence is wisdom in acting rightly. The best action is often to win the games you play, but the prudent human being may sometimes find losing to be the right thing. Block's deed is an act of prudence, insofar as it conduces not to his own preservation, but to the good life in general. The melancholy knight sacrifices himself and those about him so that a child may grow and a family may flourish. No act can be more disinterested, and Immanuel Kant says that disinterestedness is the central element of right moral action. Despite his insistence on his alienation from and indifference toward other humans, the world-weary Block proves capable of great selfless *charity*.

In *The City of God*, St. Augustine writes, "When a man's purpose is to love God not according to man, but according to God, and to love his neighbor as himself, he is beyond doubt said to be of good will because of this love. This disposition is more usually called 'charity' [*caritas*] in Holy Scripture; but, in the same sacred writings, it is also called love [*amor*]."[17] Commenting on Corinthians, he also writes, "Without charity, [knowledge] puffs up: that is, it lifts us up with a pride which is only an inflated emptiness. In the demons, then, there is knowledge without charity."[18] Antonius Block yearns for knowledge—namely, the knowledge of God and how best to love Him. This never presents itself, and yet he loves his neighbor regardless. He ultimately chooses charity *without* knowledge. To do so is the rejection of the demonic, which proves to be victory over Death itself.

The relationship between things human and divine is the oldest question of philosophy, stretching back earlier than Pythagoras. The problems of the meaningful deed and the self-justification of life are literary questions, posed in a cinematic parable. The viewer of this movie can find in it the influence of the existential thinkers Bergman so voraciously read: Dostoevsky, Balzac, Flaubert, Nietzsche, Strindberg.[19] Block's charitable deed is Nietzschean in character, and he himself is "a human being who justifies

17 St. Augustine of Hippo, *The City of God against the Pagans* trans. R. W. Dyson (New York: Cambridge University Press, 1998), XIV.vii.

18 Ibid., IX.xxi.

19 See Bergman, *Magic Lantern*, 112.

man *himself*; a human being who is a stroke of luck, completing and redeeming man, and for whose sake one may hold fast to *belief in man*!"[20] With God absent, Block is a man who justifies man. The influence of Camus is also evident. Bergman greatly admired the novelist, and was once close to adapting Camus' *The Fall* for the screen. Block's persistence in competing with an opponent he cannot beat is reminiscent of the labors of Sisyphus.

Today, few of us are knights or jugglers. We do not play chess with Death, except by way of strained metaphor. Nevertheless, all fables are simply true, and we can learn much from Antonius Block. Amidst the scourge of a pandemic, we do not hear the voice of God. Nor are our fabricated replacements for the divine—the state, the technicians, the "authorities"—able to guide us or invest our suffering with meaning. We are thrown back on our own wit to discover what it means to live well in times of plague. It remains possible to reject this assignment, and to give ourselves over to fearful superstition. Many people are able to understand suffering only as retaliation for iniquity. We may whip ourselves and others in the streets or, more commonly, we may load up scapegoats with the sins of the tribe. The natural candidates are the same politicians, technicians, and authorities that we once set up as idols and by whom we now feel abandoned. Such responses are driven by passion, and show clearly that sound reasoning has been subordinated to fear.

The charitable sacrifice is what prudence demands, *not* the irrational and magical sacrifice. The deeds that redeem humanity when God turns away are deeds of charity. To love our neighbors and give succor to those in need invests human life with meaning and purpose. This meaning is self-generated, and is a victory of the will. Fear in the face of plague is natural, but fear must not pilot the organism. Wisdom must always guide fear. Self-scourging penitence negates the intrinsic value of human life. Ours cannot and need not be the total sacrifice of Block, but hazarding the risk of infection when lending a hand to another would be a great relief is still a redeeming sacrifice. It affirms humanity from within rather than waiting on external affirmation. The good life is the domain of thoughtful *caritas*.

20 Friedrich Nietzsche, *On the Genealogy of Morality*, trans. Alan J. Swenson and Maudemarie Clark (Indianapolis: Hackett, 1998), 24.

CHAPTER X

José Saramago

Blindness

Flourishing Requires Community

Throughout this work, I have discussed the classical idea of prudence and its connection to the good life. These are expressions taken from the ethical writing of Aristotle. For Aristotle, prudence is wisdom in right action, and right action is that which most conduces to happiness. The prudent human being can successfully deliberate on what behaviors and actions are appropriate in particular situations for achieving the best outcomes. Outcomes are measured in reference to happiness, and the good life is the happiest life.

"Happiness" here is an imprecise translation of Aristotle's word, *eudaimonia.* This literally means "having a good daimon," or living one's life under the guidance of a beneficent spirit. Socrates speaks often of his "daimon," the inner voice that guides his decisions at important moments. Aristotle calls *eudaimonia* the highest of all goods. He writes, "Both the general run of men and people of superior refinement say that [the highest good] is happiness (*eudaimonia*), and identify living well and faring well with being happy; but with regard to what happiness is they differ."[1] The good life, the life of happiness, consists of *living well* and *faring well*. Prudence aims at living well, while faring well is subject to chance. *Eudaimonia* is, as Aristotle's translators note, "more than a sentiment or feeling, more than the pleasure of the moment or even a series of satisfied desires. *Eudaimonia* ... encompasses the excellence specific to human beings as human beings—what Aristotle famously calls 'virtue.'"[2] A better translation of *eudaimonia* is "flourishing." Flourishing refers not to any momentary gratification, but to a holistic condition of life.

Aristotle's *eudaimonia* is not a doctrine of egoism or solipsism. He writes, "While making has an end other than itself, action cannot; for good action itself is its end. It is for this reason that we think Pericles and men like him have practical wisdom, viz. because they can see what is good for

---

1 Aristotle, *Nic. Eth.*, I.iv.1095a17–20.

2 Robert C. Bartlett and Susan D. Collins, Translators' Introduction to *Aristotle's Nicomachean Ethics* (Chicago: University of Chicago Press, 2012), x.

themselves and what is good for men in general."[3] Right action is not the same as utilitarian or expedient action. It does not aim only at a particular, circumstantial good, nor does it look only to the private good of the individual. For Aristotle, the idea of a wholly private good is spurious. The individual cannot flourish unless his or her society also flourishes. Happiness requires good socio-political conditions. This is why, while Socrates and Plato often suggest that retreating from the political sphere is a prerequisite for the philosopher to live well, Aristotle takes political engagement to be a necessity of the human condition. He writes, "It is evident that the state is a creation of nature, and that man is by nature a political animal. And he who by nature and not by mere accident is without a state is either a bad man or above humanity."[4]

The pristine spirit that transcends all bodily conditions and honors its virtue over its life is the ideal of the Stoics. However, a complete human life requires more than just a good death. True flourishing as a human being is contingent upon both one's own virtue and character, and also the conditions of one's society. The individual and society depend on one another for prosperity. If the average character of the people in one's community is vicious and depraved, and there is not a culture of mutual respect and co-dependence, the highest degrees of *eudaimonia* will be unattainable. If society is overrun with an *ethos* of expedience, and each member seeks only his or her private good, the effect is counter-purposive. The level of happiness one can achieve in such an egoistic society is severely limited. Nations of this type lack good laws, good infrastructure, economic stability, and so forth. The autocrat must live in constant fear and vexation. Only in societies that work together to achieve common goals, and set aside private interest when demanded by the public good, is flourishing truly possible. In the moral philosophy of Cicero, therefore, public virtue always transcends private virtue: "The duties prescribed by justice must be given precedence over the pursuit of knowledge and the duties imposed by it; for the former concern the welfare of our fellow-men; and nothing ought to be more sacred in men's eyes than that."[5]

To properly speak of prudence, we must speak of practical wisdom that conduces to the good for all human beings. Aristotle calls the form of human wit that is skillful at attaining private ends "cleverness," and he cautions that "if the mark be noble, the cleverness is laudable, but if the

---

3 Aristotle, *Nic. Eth.*, VI.v.1140b6-10.
4 Aristotle, *Pol.*, I.ii.1253a2-4.
5 Cicero, *On Duties*, I.xliii.155.

mark be bad, the cleverness is mere villainy."[6] Cleverness is a knack for problem-solving, but without the direction of wisdom it does not lead one to the good life. A state of flourishing requires a practical wisdom that looks to the good of the whole, and it requires a fully developed spirit of community.

Aristotle's notion of *eudaimonia* is particularly relevant in times of crisis. The pandemic that disrupts the psychological and physical life of a people, like the war that decimates a nation's land and population, is a public evil. It harms all individuals within a community, although not all in the same way or to the same degree. A sudden financial reversal or the death of a loved one is a private evil. The sufferer may receive compassion from friends, but the weight of the loss itself does not fall on these friends. With public evils, an entire community is disrupted and oppressed by misfortune, and each member bears a weight similar to that of others.

The clever individual may be able to turn pandemics to profit. Timely investments in emerging technologies, or the controlled distribution of community needs can yield a great deal of personal gain. Villains often use their cleverness to exploit fear and shortage, conning desperate persons and further aggravating the general crisis. For humans to truly flourish in times of pandemics, however, right action is necessary. What will it profit a man if he gain a fortune, but destroys civilization in order to do so? Right action in this case is action that conduces to the good life for the entire community. Justice, equity, and other social virtues are particularly important in crisis situations.

In order to flourish during pandemics, it is imperative that communities work together. This is the lesson taught by José Saramago (1922–2010) in his 1995 novel, *Blindness*. Saramago was a distinguished Portuguese writer, and the recipient of the 1998 Nobel Prize for Literature. In its announcement of the award, the Nobel committee cited *Blindness*, among other works. Harold Bloom wrote that Saramago, along with Octavio Paz, was one of the only recent winners "who conferred honor upon that award," and he also stated in 2002 that Saramago "seems to me the most gifted novelist alive in the world today."[7] The relationship of the human condition to morbidity and mortality was a constant theme throughout Saramago's writing, and it reaches its finest expression in *Blindness*.[8]

---

6 Aristotle, *Nic. Eth.*, VI.xii.1144a25-27.

7 Harold Bloom, *Genius*, 537; 596.

8 See also José Saramago, *Death with Interruptions*, trans. Margaret Jull Costa (New York: Mariner Books, 2009), which begins, "The following day, no one died. This fact,

Blindness is a dark novel about a fictional pandemic that affects the entire population of an unnamed nation, and possibly beyond. None of the characters of the novel are given proper names, as the pandemic effaces all personal identities. The only symptom of the disease is total white blindness, and it strikes immediately, without warning. The story begins with patient zero, who emerges from an automobile stopped in traffic to announce, "I am blind" (2).[9] From this character, "the first blind man," the disease spreads to all those who encounter him: his wife, an opportunistic thief who steals his car, the ophthalmologist who analyzes his ailment, the other patients in the doctor's office (a young prostitute called "the girl with the dark glasses"; "the old man with the black eyepatch"; "the boy with the squint"). Soon, the civic authorities have taken notice of the outbreak, and take severe steps to isolate and contain the infected. These seven persons, along with the wife of the doctor, are the first eight patients admitted to an abandoned asylum, converted quickly into a pest-house for the purpose of containment. The doctor's wife is the only character who, for unknown reasons, retains her sight throughout the narrative, but her loyalty to her husband compels her to feign blindness in order to tend to him during the quarantine.

At first, food is left for the patients, but no doctors or nurses are willing to risk infection by coming into contact with the afflicted. Armed military personnel police the perimeter of the building to ensure no one attempts escape, and fear of infection makes the guards prone to drastic measures. Within the asylum-prison, the blind are left to govern themselves and figure out how best to live. Anonymous authorities daily repeat the same formal orders through the loudspeakers, reminding the inmates that they are effectively abandoned by the outside world. These orders have the imperative and impersonal tone of concentration camps. "Leaving the building without authorization will mean instant death … three times daily food will be deposited at the main door … all left-overs must be burnt … in the event of a fire getting out of control, either accidentally or on purpose, the firemen will not intervene … the internees cannot count on any outside intervention should there be any outbreaks of illnesses, nor in the event of any disorder or aggression … in the case of death, whatever the cause, the internees will bury the corpse in the yard without any

being absolutely contrary to life's rules, provoked enormous and in the circumstances, perfectly justifiable anxiety in people's minds" (1).

9 All parenthetical citations in this chapter refer to José Saramago, *Blindness*, trans. Giovanni Pontiero (New York: Harcourt, 1997).

formalities" (43). The detainees are left on their own to face all disturbances, of whatever nature. No physician will treat illness, no firefighter will respond to conflagration, and no police will prevent or punish criminality. These are the civic institutions most foundational for social stability. Further, the population that must go without any help is utterly blind, and cast into a foreign environment with minimal resources. To live in such a manner is to live entirely outside of organized civilization.

In Hebrew Scripture, Cain is punished for his fratricide with perpetual exile from all civil society. Yahweh tells Cain, "You will be a fugitive and a wanderer upon the earth." Cain is then branded with a mark, so that all may know his ignominy and "no one who came upon him would kill him."[10] The infected persons in *Blindness* suffer a similar fate. They are cut off from all of the benefits and public goods of society. Abandoned by law and social order, they enter into a state of nature. "We all heard the orders," says the doctor. "Whatever happens now, one thing we can be sure of, no one will come to our assistance, therefore we ought to start getting organized without delay" (45). However, while the doctor envisions the ratification of a social contract, the unrestrained license of statelessness quickly prevails.

The state of nature portrayed by Saramago is that of Thomas Hobbes' *Leviathan*. Hobbes writes, "It is manifest, that during the time men live without a common power to keep them all in awe, they are in that condition which is called war, and such a war, as is of every man, against every man." Unfettered by the superior violence of transcendental authority, the natural condition of human beings is a war of all against all. Hobbes continues, "In such condition, there is … continual fear, and danger of violent death; and the life of man, solitary, poor, nasty, brutish, and short." Under such conditions, "this also is consequent; that nothing can be unjust. The notions of right and wrong, justice and injustice have there no place. Where there is no common power, there is no law: where no law, no injustice. Force, and fraud, are in war the two cardinal virtues."[11] The first act of aggression in *Blindness* is sexual: the car thief fondles the breast of the prostitute. She responds with a swift kick, and her stiletto punctures the thief's thigh. With no medical aid forthcoming, his leg becomes infected, and when he ventures outside to ask the guards for help, he is unceremoniously gunned down: "The face of a blind man. Fear made the soldier's

---

10 Gen. 4:12; 4:15.

11 Thomas Hobbes, *Leviathan*, ed. J. C. A. Gaskin (New York: Oxford University Press, 1996), 84–85.

blood freeze, and fear drove him to aim his weapon and release a blast of gunfire at close range" (75).

After this, social conditions progressively worsen within the asylum, as more and more inmates are introduced, filling the building well beyond capacity. Hobbes' analysis of the state of nature is not a perfect parallel to the situation in *Blindness*. The Hobbesian state of nature precedes all social forms. It is there at the beginning, coming before the development of civil states. People in the state of nature are wretched, but they are all equally well equipped to survive. The law of nature—that is, the law of total war—is the air they breathe and the only *ethos* they know. In Saramago's narrative, human beings are thrust from a fully developed civilization, where they are habituated to think and act in terms of justice and good order, into a lawless state of nature, which is for them an utterly foreign *Umwelt*. Hobbes' narrative must be supplemented by observations from two other philosophers. The first is Jean-Jacques Rousseau's assertion that, were a modern human being to be suddenly uprooted and thrown into the state of nature, he or she would be unable to survive very long. Rousseau writes, "In becoming habituated to the ways of society and a slave, [the modern human] becomes weak, fearful, and servile; his soft and effeminate lifestyle completes the enervation of both his strength and his courage."[12]

Secondly, Giambattista Vico observes that there are two distinct forms of barbarism, the "barbarism of sense" and the "barbarism of reflection." He writes, "Through long centuries of barbarism, rust will consume the misbegotten subtleties of malicious wits that have turned them into beasts made more inhuman by the barbarism of reflection than the first men had been made by the barbarism of sense. For the latter displayed a generous savagery, against which one could defend oneself or take flight or be on one's guard; but the former, with a base savagery, under soft words and embraces, plots against the life and fortune of friends and intimates." In pre-social times, barbarians have only sensation as their guide. Their weapon is physical force, which they use to terrorize others, but this can be countered by equal violence. The barbarian of reflection is of a different sort. Such a person, "with a base savagery, under soft words and embraces, plots against the life and fortune of friends and intimates."[13] The cultured barbarian of today is not a rampaging brute, but cunning and manipulative; he robs others with a pen rather than a club. The barbarian of

---

12 Jean-Jacques Rousseau, *Discourse on the Origin of Inequality*, in *The Basic Political Writings*, trans. Donald A. Cress (Indianapolis: Hackett, 1987), 43.

13 Vico, *New Science*, §1106.

reflection cannot be guarded against, and reaps far more destruction than his predecessors. The brute barbarian can only harm those unfortunates within the range of his club, but the barbarian of reflection can organize a Holocaust.

Once the asylum in *Blindness* is flooded with detainees, a dichotomy arises between the civilized and law-abiding folk, who are jarringly displaced into a strange land, and those who have long lived outside of the rule of law and the morality of justice. The criminal class of individuals is much better prepared to dominate under the conditions of the state of nature than the community of upstanding persons. The criminal has had a lifetime of training in lawlessness and the rule of force. True to Rousseau's observations, the innocent are helpless against the children of Cain. These criminals are not, however, the brute barbarians of sense of the prehistoric world, but the barbarians of reflection of today. They are armed with guns rather than clubs, and their malice extends beyond the immediate desires of the body to a systematic program of terrorism.

The criminal cadre that forms within the asylum begins by taking control of the food supply. Their source of power is the threat of violence. As the armed party, they are the superior force. "Let it be known and there is no turning back," the delinquent with the gun commands, "that from today onwards we shall take charge of the food, you've all been warned" (139). The law enforcers outside the building are deaf to the pleas of the inmates for aid. Once the criminal group has control of the food, they use it as leverage for extorting from the other inmates all of their possessions of any value. As soon as there is nothing left with which to pay, the criminals demand sexual favors. The women of the asylum are forced into sex slavery, and the most graphic abuses and degradations are described. One woman drops dead after the first experience of this barbaric rape, and the doctor's wife calls "the suddenly dislocated body" of the victim "the image of the body of all the women here" (182). The husbands of these women must accept these conditions or starve.

The basic human dignity of the innocent is utterly forsaken by the criminals and the world at large. This continues until one victimized woman, regardless of her life, burns down the asylum, with the delinquents trapped in a barricaded room. When the blind emerge, helpless and dispirited, they find no guards, and no source of authority whatsoever. "The gate is wide open, the madmen escape" (216). The entire nation has been exposed to the contagion, and everyone is now blind. All of the necessary institutions of civic life have halted. There is no food production, no government, and no help forthcoming. There is only a city of ghosts groping for survival day to day.

Saramago has imagined a worst case scenario for a pandemic. In his model, the entire framework of civilization is dissolved. In spite of this, the book in *not* pessimistic. Despite the ghastly conditions, the central characters are able to survive the outbreak and find a modicum of happiness by forming their own mutually beneficial society. The first blind man and his wife, the girl with the dark glasses, the boy, the old man with the eye patch, the doctor, and the doctor's wife (the one person remaining who is able to see) become an insular tribe. Saramago writes, "They stay together, pressed up against each other, like a flock, no one there wants to be the lost sheep, for they know that no shepherd will come looking for them" (217). It is only by cooperation and sacrifice that this group is able to outlast the pestilence.

In the Hobbesian world that this group emerges into, the rule of behavior is self-preservation. The blind no longer know how to find their own homes, so they wander like Bedouins, groping around, hoping to stumble onto food. All other human beings are rivals for the limited resources of the city. Mere existence is a contest of all against all. Civilization descends to the worst sort of barbarism, in which no social ties whatsoever are recognized. When families become separated, parents and children, husbands and wives wander off alone, with no means of finding the others. Should they meet again, there will be no recognition; they will meet as ravenous beasts competing for a shank of meat. The city becomes a jungle, in which *strength* is the only rule of justice. Because the survival of one is predicated on the misfortune of all others, every human interaction is a battle, bearing a violent character. Those unwilling to risk their lives are doomed to death by starvation. At best, urbane men and women are reduced to life in "primitive hordes … with the difference that we are not a few thousand men and women in an immense, unspoiled nature, but thousands of millions in an uprooted, exhausted world" (256).

There are two Latin proverbs concerning the relationship of one human being to another, *homo homini Deus* and *homo homini lupus*, on which Hobbes reflects in the dedication of his *De cive*. He writes, "To speak impartially, both sayings are very true: that *man to man is a kind of God*; and that *man to man is an arrant wolf*."[14] The solitary individuals that encounter one another in the streets of the city do not deserve the

14 Thomas Hobbes, *The Citizen*, in *Man and Citizen*, ed. Bernard Gert (Indianapolis: Hackett, 1991), 89.

appellative "human," for they are united by no shared projects and no sense of sympathy. They are to one another two beasts of prey meeting over a carcass in a wasteland. This antisocial behavior promises only a life that is, as Hobbes says, "solitary, poor, nasty, brutish, and short." The doctor's wife discovers a storeroom in the basement of a grocery store that still contains chickpeas and various canned goods, and accidentally tips off blind scavengers to its existence. When she returns to gather more provisions, the basement is full of rotting corpses, the stench overwhelming. "They must have found the basement," she laments, "rushed down the stairs looking for food … and if one fell, they would all fall, they probably never reached where they wanted to go, or if they did they could not turn because of the obstruction on the staircase … Most likely other blind people closed [the door], converting the basement into an enormous tomb and I am to blame for what happened" (314). In their egoistic greed for survival, the wolves trample and claw one another to death. This attitude of hostility leads to mutually assured destruction. Without social instincts, without the rule of human decency, none lend a hand to others, and all suffer.

The central group, on the other hand, recognizes the need for cooperation. By banding together, they become as gods one to another. The self-sacrifice of any one member for the good of the group makes life more bearable for the group as a whole. They prove that compassion conduces more to survival than avarice. The doctor's wife counsels, "If we stay together we might manage to survive, if we separate we shall be swallowed up by the masses and destroyed" (256). Recognizing the strength in organization, they construct a rudimentary social contract between themselves. The doctor's wife is given authority, as "a kind of natural leader, a king with eyes in the land of the blind." They establish a fixed abode in the apartment of the doctor and his wife, rather than living nomadically. The old man even insists, for the good of the group, that "when I start becoming an impossible burden, you must tell me, and if, out of friendship or pity, you should decide to say nothing, I hope I'll have enough judgment to do the necessary. … Withdraw, take myself off, disappear, as elephants used to do" (256–58).

The relations between the members of this group evolve into those of a family. The family is the basic political unit of human society. As Aristotle says, "The family is the association established by nature for the supply of men's everyday wants, and the members of it are called by

Charondas, 'companions of the cupboard.'"[15] The family is a city in brief, a group of individuals that work in unison for the good of the whole. The relationships are all personal and immediate. Brother works for the good of sister, and mother for the good of son. The family is a true community. In broader political groups, the word "community" is often inapplicable. The word "society" suggests the more impersonal ties of states and nations. The good king works in the abstract for the good of the whole, but he does not know his subjects personally. King and peasant do not share a cupboard. All subjects have their own aims and projects, their own unique ideas of the good life. In a family, there is a shared vision of good life, and right action among its members conduces to this one ideal.

The young prostitute becomes a stand-in mother figure for the boy with the squint, the fate of whose biological family is unknown. In a moment of weakness while in the asylum, she and the doctor sleep together. Rather than driving her and the doctor's wife apart, this becomes the impetus for a sort of kinship: "You have become almost like a sister, perhaps because my husband slept with you" (253). The doctor's wife, as the only member of the family with sight, often shows a maternalism toward her husband, who is the most learned and logical of the group, but who is as helpless as any without his vision. The old man with the eye patch and the young girl with dark glasses become lovers, and declare themselves bound in symbolic solemn matrimony. "We'll start living together here, like a couple, and we shall continue living together if we have to separate from our friends, two blind people must be able to see more than one" (306). These sorts of bonds are more than the bonds of basic decorum that abide between strangers thrown together by chance. These are the bonds of kinship, bonds of the deepest fidelity and compassion.

In the end, the term of the pandemic passes and sight is restored to the characters. The pestilence comes and goes without explanation. The doctor muses cryptically, "I don't think we did go blind, I think we are blind, Blind but seeing, Blind people who can see, but do not see" (326). We go through life with all of our faculties, yet we lack prudence. We do not apprehend the good life, however well we may see. We do not live rightly, and to that extent we are already blind.

The good life requires community. It requires restraining our self-interest and our private passions and working in accord with our neighbors. The person who renounces community is Cain, a fugitive in the wilderness. Cain can survive, he can dominate others, and he can attain wealth and

15 Aristotle, *Pol.*, I.ii.1252b13–15.

power. However, he can never truly flourish. To flourish requires full membership in a community that is also flourishing. Cain succeeds through the exploitation and oppression of other human beings, and his success is has the character of arbitrary license. However successful he may be, Cain is always blind. As Saramago's prostitute wisely observes, two blind people can always see more than one, three more than two, and so on.

Saramago's lesson is of the utmost importance today. We are counseled to support one another during times of pandemic. We are counseled to sacrifice our own petty self-interest for the sake of community. It is not the time to ask what we can gain by this crisis. Profiteering renders the whole world worse off, and one's own capacity for flourishing is undermined by a world gone mad. American politicians with foreknowledge of COVID-19 were quick to sell off their stocks and invest in communications technology. Charlatans have dramatically over-charged desperate public leaders for needed medical equipment. Average citizens have rushed to overstock on common staple items, creating national shortages. What is the nature of these people's "prosperity"? They have demonstrated cleverness, but not prudence. They have renounced community for the sake of barbarism, and barbarism is a state of total war.

Prudence demands investment in one's community. Crises upset the equilibrium of a nation. The good life can only be attained when society rebounds and social institutions once more operate as they ought. To support this process is to act toward one's own *eudaimonia*. The greater one's ties to a flourishing community, the more one is capable of flourishing oneself. To act contrary to the public good is acting against the possibility of *eudaimonia*. A world in which men and women shoot at those who plead for aid, or trample one another in their race for chickpeas is an impoverished world. Saramago shows that even in a world full of wolves it is better to be gods to one another.

HONORABLE MENTION

The works mentioned above reflect the interests of the author more than any other considerations. There are many other works that merit consideration. Below are a few further books the curious reader might enjoy.

Margaret Atwood, *Oryx and Crake* trilogy (*Oryx and Crake*, 2003; *The Year of the Flood*, 2009; *MaddAddam*, 2013).

Geraldine Brooks, *Year of Wonders*, 2001.

Geoffrey Chaucer, *Canterbury Tales*, "Pardoner's Tale," c. 1392.

John Dos Passos, *The Big Money*, "Mary French," 1936.

Homer, *The Iliad*, Book I, 12th or 13th Century BCE.

Eugène Ionesco, *Rhinoceros*, 1959.

Tony Kushner, *Angels in America*, 1991–92.

Jean de La Fontaine, "The Animals Sick of the Plague," c. 1668.

Jack London, *The Scarlet Plague*, 1912.

Naguib Mahfouz, *The Harafish*, 1977.

Emily St. John Mandel, *Station Eleven*, , 2014.

W. Somerset Maugham, *The Painted Veil*, 1925.

Gabriel García Márquez, *Love in the Time of Cholera*, 1985.

Thomas Nashe, "Litany in the Time of Plague," 1592.

Francesco Petrarca, *Letters on Familiar Matters* VIII, 7 and 8, c. 1353.

Edgar Allen Poe, "The Masque of the Red Death," 1842.

Katherine Anne Porter, *Pale Horse, Pale Rider*, 1939.

Procopius of Caesarea, *History of the Wars*, Book II, c. 553.

Philip Roth, *Nemesis*, 2010.

Lucius Annaeus Seneca, *Oedipus*, 1st Century CE.

Mary Shelley, *The Last Man*, 1826.

John Wilson, "The City of the Plague," 1816.

BIBLIOGRAPHY

Adorno, Theodor W. *Prisms*. Trans. Samuel and Shierry Weber. Cambridge, MA: The MIT Press, 1983.

Ali, Abdullah Yusuf, trans. *The Holy Qur'an*. Hertfordshire: Wordsworth, 2000.

Aristotle. *The Complete Works of Aristotle*. 2 vols. Ed. Jonathan Barnes. Princeton, NJ: Princeton University Press, 1984.

St. Augustine of Hippo. *The City of God against the Pagans*. Trans. R. W. Dyson. New York: Cambridge University Press, 1998.

Barfield, Raymond. *The Ancient Quarrel between Philosophy and Poetry*. New York: Cambridge University Press, 2011.

Bartlett, Robert C., and Susan D. Collins. Translators' Introduction to *Aristotle's Nicomachean Ethics*. Chicago: University of Chicago Press, 2012.

Bataille, Georges. *The Absence of Myth*. Trans. Michael Richardson. New York: Verso, 1994.

Beckett, Samuel. *Murphy*. New York: Grove Press, 1957.

———. *Three Novels*. New York: Grove Weidenfeld, 1991.

St. Benedict of Nursia. *St. Benedict's Rule for Monasteries*. Trans. Leonard J. Doyle. Collegeville, MN: The Liturgical Press, 1950.

Benjamin, Walter. *The Work of Art in the Age of Its Technological Reproducibility and Other Writings on Media*. Trans. Edmund Jephcott et al. Cambridge, MA: Belknap Press, 2008.

Bergman, Ingmar. *The Magic Lantern: An Autobiography*. Trans. Joan Tate. Chicago: University of Chicago Press, 2007.

———, dir. *The Seventh Seal* [*Det sjunde inseglet*]. Stockholm: Svensk Filmindustri, 1957.

Bertherat, Eric et al. "Plague Reappearance in Algeria after 50 Years, 2003." *Emerging Infectious Diseases* 13 (Oct. 2007): 1459–62

Bloom, Harold. *Genius: A Mosaic of One Hundred Exemplary Creative Minds*. New York: Warner Books, 2002.

Boccaccio, Giovanni. *The Decameron*. Trans. G. H. McWilliam. New York: Penguin, 1972.

Bolotin, David. "Thucydides." In *History of Political Philosophy*, ed. Leo Strauss and Joseph Cropsey. Chicago: University of Chicago Press, 1987, 7–32.

Botton, Alain de. "Camus on the Coronavirus." *The New York Times* (19 Mar. 2020).

Bragg, Melvyn. *The Seventh Seal*. London: British Film Institute, 1993.

Brant, Sebastian. *The Ship of Fools*. Trans. Edwin H. Zeydel. New York: Columbia University Press, 1944.

Brée, Germaine. "Albert Camus and the Plague." *Yale French Studies* 8 (1951): 93–100.

———, ed. *Camus: A Collection of Critical Essays*. Englewood Cliffs, NJ: Prentice-Hall, 1962.

Burckhardt, Jacob. *The Civilization of the Renaissance in Italy*. Trans. S. G. C. Middlemore, rev. Ludwig Goldscheider. New York: Modern Library, 1995.

Burt, Daniel S. *The Novel 100*. New York: Checkmark, 2004.

Camus, Albert. *Caligula and 3 Other Plays*. Trans. Stuart Gilbert. New York: Random House, 1958.

———. *The Myth of Sisyphus and Other Essays*. Trans. Justin O'Brien. New York: Vintage, 1955.

———, *The Plague*. Trans. Stuart Gilbert. New York: Modern Library, 1948.

———. *The Stranger*. Trans. Matthew Ward. New York: Vintage, 1989.

Cassirer, Ernst. *Language and Myth.* Trans. Susanne K. Langer. New York: Dover, 1946.

———. *The Myth of the State.* New Haven, CT: Yale University Press, 1973.

———. *The Philosophy of Symbolic Forms.* 3 vols. Trans. Ralph Manheim. New Haven, CT: Yale University Press, 1955.

Cawley, A. C., ed. *Everyman and Medieval Miracle Plays.* New York: E. P. Dutton & Co., 1959.

Cicero, Marcus Tullius. *On Duties.* Trans. Walter Miller. Cambridge, MA: Harvard University Press, 1913.

———. *De inventione.* Trans. H. M. Hubbell. Cambridge, MA: Harvard University Press, 1949.

———. *De natura Deorum.* Trans. H. Rackham. Cambridge, MA: Harvard University Press, 1979.

Collingwood, R. G. *An Essay on Philosophical Method.* Bristol: Thoemmes, 1995.

Coogan, Michael D., ed. *The New Oxford Annotated Bible.* New York: Oxford, 2001.

Copenhaver, Brian P., and Charles B. Schmitt. *Renaissance Philosophy.* New York: Oxford University Press, 1992.

Croce, Benedetto. *History, Its Theory and Practice.* Trans. Douglas Ainslie. New York: Harcourt, Brace and Co., 1921.

Defoe, Daniel. *A Journal of the Plague Year.* New York: Signet, 1960.

———. *Robinson Crusoe.* New York: Bantam, 1981.

Descartes, Réne. *The Philosophical Writings of Descartes.* 3 vols. Trans. John Cottingham, Robert Stoothoff, and Dugald Murdoch. New York: Cambridge University Press, 1997.

Dilthey, Wilhelm. *Selected Works, vol. 5: Poetry and Experience*. Ed. Rudolf A Makkreel and Frithjof Rodi. Princeton, NJ: Princeton University Press, 1985.

Durkheim, Émile. *Suicide*. Trans. John A Spaulding and George Simpson. New York: Free Press, 1979.

Ebert, Roger. *The Great Movies*. New York: Broadway Books, 2002.

Eco, Umberto. *The Name of the Rose*. Trans. William Weaver. New York: Harcourt Brace & Company, 1984.

———. *Six Walks in the Fictional Woods.* Cambridge, MA: Harvard University Press, 1995.

———. *The Story of the Betrothed.* Trans. Stephen Sartarelli, ill. Marcoi Lorenzetti. London: Pushkin Children's Books, 2017.

———. *Travels in Hyperreality*. Trans. William Weaver. New York: Harcourt Brace & Company, 1986.

Eliot, T. S. *The Complete Plays and Poems: 1909–1950*. New York: Harcourt, Brace & World, 1962.

Epictetus. *The Discourses*. In *Discourses and Selected Writings*, trans. and ed. Robert Dobbin. New York: Penguin, 2008.

Euripides. *The Bacchae*. Trans. William Arrowsmith. In *Euripides V*, ed. David Grene and Richmond Lattimore. Chicago: University of Chicago Press, 1968.

Ficino, Marsilio. *Platonic Theology*. 6 vols. Trans. Michael J. B. Allen. Cambridge, MA: Harvard University Press, 2006.

Fletcher, Robert. *A Tragedy of the Great Plague of Milan in 1630*. Baltimore: The Lord Baltimore Press, 1898.

Flynn, Thomas R. *Existentialism: A Very Short Introduction*. New York: Oxford University Press, 2006.

Foucault, Michel. *Discipline and Punish*. Trans. Alan Sheridan. New York: Vintage, 1995.

Galen, Aelius. *On the Natural Faculties*. Trans. Arthur John Brock. Cambridge, MA: Harvard University Press, 2006.

Goethe, Johann Wolfgang von. *The Poems of Goethe*. Trans. E. A. Browning et al. New York: Thomas Y. Crowell & Co., 1882.

Guarino, Guido A. Introduction to *On Famous Women* (Giovanni Boccaccio). New York: Italica Press, 2011.

Hays, J. N. *Epidemics and Pandemics: Their Impacts on Human History*. Santa Barbara, CA: ABC-Clio, 2005.

Hegel, G. W. F. *Phenomenology of Spirit*. Trans. A. V. Miller. New York: Oxford University Press, 1977.

Hesiod. *Works and Days*. Trans. Richmond Lattimore. Ann Arbor, MI: University of Michigan Press, 1991.

Hobbes, Thomas. *Leviathan*. Ed. J. C. A. Gaskin. New York: Oxford University Press, 1996.

———. *Man and Citizen*. Ed. Bernard Gert. Indianapolis: Hackett, 1991.

Homer. *The Iliad*. Trans. Robert Fagles. New York: Penguin, 1998.

Honigsbaum, Mark. *The Pandemic Century: One Hundred Years of Panic, Hysteria, and Hubris* New York: W. W. Norton, 2019.

Hyde, Lewis. *Trickster Makes this World*. New York: Farras, Straus & Giroux, 1988.

James, William. *Principles of Psychology*. 2 vols. New York: Dover, 1950.

Jung, Carl. *The Archetypes and the Collective Unconscious*. Trans. R. F. C. Hull. Princeton, NJ: Princeton University Press, 1990.

Kelly, John. *The Great Mortality*. New York: HarperCollins, 2005.

Kierkegaard, Søren. *Fear and Trembling*. Trans. Howard V. Hong and Edna H. Hong. Princeton, NJ: Princeton University Press, 1983.

———. *Philosophical Fragments*. Trans. Howard V. Hong and Edna H. Hong. Princeton, NJ: Princeton University Press, 1985.

Kristeller, Paul Oskar. *Renaissance Thought*. New York: Harper & Row, 1961.

Kundera, Milan. *The Book of Laughter and Forgetting*. Trans. Aaron Asher. New York: HarperPerennial, 1999.

Landon, William J. *Lorenzo di Filippo Strozzi and Niccolò Machiavelli: Patron, Client, and the* Pistola fatta per la peste. Toronto: University of Toronto Press, 2013.

Lipsius, Justus. *On Constancy*. Trans. Sir John Stradling, ed. John Sellars. Exeter: Bristol Phoenix Press, 2006.

Littman, Robert J. "The Plague of Athens: Epidemiology and Paleopathology." *Mount Sinai Journal of Medicine* 76 (2009): 456–67.

London, Jack. *The Scarlet Plague*. New York: Macmillan, 1915.

Lowenstein, Roger. "In Camus' 'The Plague,' lessons about fear, quarantine and the human spirit." *The Washington Post* (3 Apr. 2020).

Lucian of Samosata. *Selected Dialogues*. Trans. C. D. N. Costa. New York: Oxford University Press, 2009.

Machiavelli, Niccolò. *The Art of War*. Trans. Ellis Farneworth, rev. Neal Wood. Cambridge, MA: Da Capo, 2001.

———. Florentine *Histories*. Trans. Laura F. Banfield and Harvey C. Mansfield, Jr. Princeton, NJ: Princeton University Press, 1988.

———. *The Prince*. Trans. Harvey C. Mansfield. Chicago: University of Chicago Press, 1998.

Mann, Thomas. *Death in Venice and Seven Other Stories*. Trans. H. T. Lowe-Porter. New York: Vintage, 1989.

———. *Letters of Thomas Mann, 1889–1955*. Trans. Richard and Clara Winston. Los Angeles: University of California Press, 1975.

———. *The Magic Mountain*. Trans. H. T. Lowe-Porter. New York: Alfred A. Knopf, 1946.

Manzoni, Alessandro. *The Betrothed.* Trans. Archibald Colquhoun. New York: E. P. Dutton & Co., 1961.

———. *On the Historical Novel.* Trans. Sandra Bermann. Lincoln, NE: University of Nebraska Press, 1984.

Marlowe, Christopher. *The Jew of Malta.* Ed. David Bevington. Manchester: Manchester University Press, 1997.

McLuhan, Marshall. *Understanding Media: The Extensions of Man.* New York: Signet, 1966.

Merleau-Ponty, Maurice. *Sense and Non-Sense.* Trans. Hubert L. Dreyfus and Patricia Allen Dreyfus. Evanston, IL: Northwestern University Press, 1964.

Metcalf, Stephen. "Albert Camus' 'The Plague' and our own Great Reset." *Los Angeles Times* (23 Mar. 2020).

Micek, John L. "In resolution, Pa. lawmaker blames COVID-19 outbreak on 'our presumptuous sins.'" *The Philadelphia Tribune* (24 Mar. 2020).

Mitchell, Peta. *Contagious Metaphor.* New York: Bloomsbury, 2014.

Montaigne, Michel de. *The Complete Essays of Montaigne.* Trans. Donald M. Frame. Stanford, CA: Stanford University Press, 1976.

Morrison, Alan S., Julius Kirshner, and Anthony Molho. "Epidemics in Renaissance Florence." *American Journal of Public Health* 75 (1985): 528–35.

Mullett, Charles F. "The English plague scare of 1720–23." *Osiris* 2 (1936): 484–516

Najemy, John M. *Between Friends: Discourses of Power and Desire in the Machiavelli—Vettori Letters of 1513–1515.* Princeton, NJ: Princeton University Press, 1993.

———. *A History of Florence, 1200–1575.* Malden, MA: Blackwell, 2008.

Nicholson, Trish. *A Biography of Story, a Brief History of Humanity*. Leicestershire: Matador, 2016.

Nietzsche, Friedrich. *Beyond Good and Evil*. Trans. Walter Kaufmann. New York: Vintage, 1989.

———. *The Birth of Tragedy and The Case of Wagner*. Trans. Walter Kaufmann. New York: Vintage, 1967.

———. *On the Genealogy of Morality*. Trans. Alan J. Swenson and Maudemarie Clark. Indianapolis: Hackett, 1998.

Ortega y Gasset, José. *Meditations on Quixote*. Trans. Evelyn Rugg and Diego Marín. Urbana, IL: University of Illinois Press, 2000.

Peone, Dustin. *Making Philosophy Laugh: Humor, Irony, and Folly in Philosophical Thought*. Eugene, OR: Cascade, 2023.

———. *Memory as Philosophy: The Theory and Practice of Philosophical Recollection*. Stuttgart: ibidem, 2019.

———. *Plague Literature: Lessons for Living Well during a Pandemic*. Atlanta: Theuth, 2020.

———. *Shame, Fame, and the Technological Mentality*. Lanham, MD: Lexington, 2021.

Petrarch, Francesco. *Letters on Familiar Matters*. 3 vols. Trans. Aldo S. Bernardo. New York: Italica Press, 2005.

Pieper, Josef. *Leisure, the Basis of Culture*. Trans. Gerald Malsbary. South Bend, IN: St. Augustine Press, 1998.

Pinton, Giorgio A. *The Conspiracy of the Prince of Macchia & G. B. Vico*. New York: Rodopi, 2013.

Plato. *Complete Works*. Ed. John M. Cooper. Indianapolis: Hackett, 1997.

Popkin, Richard. *The History of Skepticism: From Savonarola to Bayle*. New York: Oxford University Press, 2003.

Proust, Marcel. *Remembrance of Things Past*. 2 vols. Trans. C. K. Scott Moncrieff and Frederick A. Blossom. New York: Random House, 1932.

Rabelais, François. *The Complete Works of François Rabelais*. Trans. Donald M. Frame. Los Angeles: University of California Press, 1999.

Rousseau, Jean-Jacques. *Discourse on the Origin of Inequality*. In *The Basic Political Writings*, trans. Donald A. Cress. Indianapolis: Hackett, 1987.

Saramago, José. *Blindness*. Trans. Giovanni Pontiero. New York: Harcourt, 1997.

———. *Death with Interruptions*. Trans. Margaret Jull Costa. New York: Mariner Books, 2009.

Sartre, Jean-Paul. *Being and Nothingness*. Trans. Hazel E. Barnes. New York: Washington Square Press, 1984.

———. *Existentialism and Human Emotions*. Trans. Hazel E. Barnes and Bernard Frechtman. New York: Philosophical Library, 1957.

Seneca, Lucius Annaeus. *Dialogues and Essays*. Trans. John Davie. New York: Oxford University Press, 2008.

———. *Oedipus*. In *Four Tragedies and Octavia*, trans. E. F. Watling. Baltimore: Penguin, 1974.

Shaftesbury, Anthony Ashley Cooper, third Earl of. *Characteristics of Men, Manners, Opinions, Times*. Ed. John M. Robertson. New York: Bobbs-Merrill, 1964.

Shakespeare, William. *The Oxford Shakespeare*. Ed. John Jowett et al. New York: Oxford University Press, 2005.

Snowden, Frank M. *Epidemics and Society*. New Haven, CT: Yale University Press, 2020.

———. *Naples in the Time of Cholera, 1884–1911*. New York: Cambridge University Press, 2002.

Sophocles. *Oedipus the King*. In *Sophocles I*, trans. David Grene. ed. D. Grene and Richmond Lattimore. Chicago: University of Chicago Press, 1991.

Thucydides. *History of the Peloponnesian War*. Trans. Rex Warner. New York: Penguin, 1985.

Todd, Olivier. *Albert Camus: A Life*. New York: Carroll & Graf, 2000.

Toren, John. Review of *Plague Literature* (D. Peone). *Rain Taxi Review of Books* 26, no. 2 (Summer 2021): 31.

Unamuno, Miguel de. *Tragic Sense of Life*. Trans. J. E. Crawford Flitch. New York: Dover, 1954.

Vico, Giambattista. *New Science*. Trans. Thomas Goddard Bergin and Max Harold Fisch. Ithaca, NY: Cornell University Press, 1988.

Vives, Juan Luis. "A Fable about Man." Trans. Nancy Lenkeith. In *The Renaissance Philosophy of Man*, ed. Ernst Cassirer, Paul Oskar Kristeller, and John Herman Randall, Jr. Chicago: University of Chicago Press, 1948, 387–93.

Zegura, Elizabeth Chesney, ed. *The Rabelais Encyclopedia*. Westport, CT: Greenwood, 2004.

Index